"The Book of Inspiring & Thought Provoking **HEALTH** Quotes."

compiled by

Scott duPont

&

Larry L. Oexner

**"The Book of
Inspiring & Thought Provoking HEALTH Quotes."**

Compiled by Scott duPont & Larry L. Oexner

Released and published by:

Nemours Publishing
c/o Nemours Marketing, Inc.
7531 Azurebrook Court
Winter Park, FL 32792
Tel: (407) 738 - 1608

ISBN # 13:978-1522715986

| U.S. | $9.99 |
| Canada | $12.99 |

Other Books in the "Inspiring Quotes" Series

Buttered Popcorn for Your Soul

Even <u>MORE</u> Inspiring Show Business Quotes

Even <u>MORE</u> of the World's Most Inspiring Quotes

*The Book of
Inspiring & Thought Provoking HEALTH Quotes*

The Greatest Book of Inspiring Quotes

The Greatest Book of Inspiring Show Business Quotes

Yet Even <u>MORE</u> of the World's Most Inspiring Quotes

Acknowledgements

We want to thank every single contributor to this book. Many of the "contributing authors" you've heard of (and probably read or heard their work), while others you may not recognize their name yet. On behalf of both of us, thank you to all of our early biology, anatomy and science teachers. We both got hooked at an early age and the fascination of science and later health inspired us to write this book to share with the world!

Also, a big thank you to Kimberly Oexner for being part of the "team" and all that you do to inspire others to get and stay healthy.

Thank YOU for getting this book! We hope you will savor and enjoy these quotes as much as we do, and share them with others as well.

Foreward

As mentioned, both of us had an early fascination with science and later health, realizing how important it is to not only live longer, but have to more energy and simply enjoy a fuller, happier life.

The idea for this book came as we were researching our latest collaboration... the book and companion documentary film: *"The Health Pill"*. Our extensive research (still continuing) from books, periodicals, medical & health journals, speeches, videos and blogs uncovered some truly inspiring quotations specifically about health. While most of the following quotes are inspiring, others are profound or thought provoking. Every single quote in this book has the power to influence you to make changes (large or small) towards better health. Even if you consider yourself a "healthy" person, there are always one or two new distinctions you can add to your lifestyle to become a better, healthier you.

Like our other "Inspiring Quotes" books, this book is meant to be slowly savored and enjoyed over time. Perhaps you keep this on your coffee table or your night stand and read a few quotes when you wake up, or before you retire to motivate you. If you find a quote that really resonates with you, we encourage you to follow that particular author and read his or her books, follow their blogs, join their YouTube channel, or attend their health seminars!

Disclaimer: while we've done our best to insure the accuracy and proper author credit for every quote, we can't guarantee with absolute certainty in the course of history (some of the quotes are hundreds of years old) who the original author is. Also, there are several doctors (M.D.'s, PhD's, etc.) and other notable titles in this book whose quotes we included. We did NOT include their "titles" or distinctions, since some of the best quotes were first written or spoken before they had earned those degrees. We also did not want to prejudice the other excellent quotes from health experts or nutritionists who have worked in their field for decades, but chose not to get a post graduate or medical degree.

We hope you enjoy, and cheers to your perfect health!

Scott duPont   *Larry L. Oexner*

"A cheerful frame of mind, reinforced by relaxation...
is the medicine that puts all ghosts of fear on the run."
- George Matthew Adams

"I'm great at a deathbed.
I've never given tranquillizers or psychiatric medicine.
I've given love and fun and creativity and passion and hope,
and these things ease suffering."
- Hunter Doherty "Patch" Adams

"In Russia most of the hospitals don't have any pain medicine,
they don't have any money.
So if you're with kids with cancer,
they can have metastases to the bone;
which some say is the worst pain a human can experience.
So a mother can be in a room with a child who hasn't stopped
screaming in five months...
eighty-five percent of the time I walk in there as a clown
they'll stop screaming."
- Hunter Doherty "Patch" Adams

"Nature tops the list of potent tranquilizers and stress reducers.
The mere sound of moving water has been shown
to lower blood pressure."
- Hunter Doherty "Patch" Adams

"Laughter releases endorphins and other natural mood elevating
and pain-killing chemicals, improves the transfer
of oxygen and nutrients to internal organs.
Laughter boosts the immune system and
helps the body fight off disease,
cancer cells as well as viral, bacterial and other infections.
Being happy is the best cure of all diseases!"
- Hunter Doherty "Patch" Adams

"Cheerfulness is the best promoter of health
and is as friendly to the mind as to the body."
- Joseph Addison

"I always take working out seriously,
but before a shoot I do extra sit ups and squats.
I also eat more vegetables and drink a ton of water,
because it really helps my skin glow."
- Lily Aldridge

"It's the little things you do and chew
that make the bigger difference"
- Luann Alemao

"Nuts are part of a healthy diet and
studies show those individuals who eat
nuts five times a week or more live longer
than those who don't."
- Luann Alemao

"A man is not rightly conditioned until he is a happy,
healthy, and prosperous being;
and happiness, health, and prosperity are the result of
a harmonious adjustment of the inner with the outer
of the man with his surroundings."
- James Allen

"A lot of women use pregnancy as an excuse
to let their bodies go, and that's the worst thing."
- Tracy Anderson

"I tell people to be thankful that Madonna is
showing that it's possible to be ageless
- people should applaud and celebrate that.
Anybody who criticizes her is just jealous!"
- Tracy Anderson

"I think it's very important to feed the body what it craves
and not be in your head about it, panicking, carrying around
some calorie-counting wheel in your bag
or something equally absurd.
I'm really not a fan of that at all."
- Tracy Anderson

"There is no quick easy way to the body you want...
commit yourself now to your workout and get started."
- Tracy Anderson

"You need to be dedicated to your workout,
whatever you choose."
- Tracy Anderson

"GOOD enough is NOT enough."
- Trevor Anderson

"EXCELLENCE is not necessarily being THE best,
but being YOUR best."
- Trevor Anderson

"It's not what you CAN'T do, but what you DON'T do."
- Trevor Anderson

"PROGRESS is a PROCESS."
- Trevor Anderson

"Keep your eyes on YOU.
It's fine to get inspired by others' physiques,
but you have to set your own personal standards.
People tend to fixate on their weaknesses, while at the same time
obsess over the strengths of others. That's a surefire way to
stay eternally frustrated. It's a healthier approach to acknowledge
your own strengths, and use them as benchmarks by which to
bring up your weaknesses. Learn to give yourself a pat on the back
for the improvements you make. Keep your eyes on YOU,
don't let the achievements of others dictate your obsessions."
- Alan Aragon

"The majority of health nuts will spend $100's a month
on useless supplements,
but won't spend a dime on actually
educating themselves on the facts about the body."
- Alan Aragon

"Missing one workout or going overboard
on the ice cream one night
(or maybe two) isn't going to cancel out
all the times you chose healthy.
It's the sum of all those small decisions that truly makes
a difference in overall health and happiness.
And just for the record, eating dessert
should never make you feel guilty.
- Alan Aragon

"Happiness is a state of activity."
- Aristotle

"It is well to be up before daybreak, for such habits contribute to health, wealth, and wisdom."
- Aristotle

"The energy of the mind is the essence of life."
- Aristotle

"The self-indulgent man craves for all pleasant things... and is led by his appetite to choose these at the cost of everything else."
- Aristotle

"We are what we repeatedly do.
Excellence, then, is not an act, but a habit."
- Aristotle

"God gave us the gift of life;
it is up to us to give ourselves the gift of living well."
- François-Marie Arouet (aka Voltaire)

"The art of medicine consists in amusing the patient while nature cures the disease."
- François-Marie Arouet (aka Voltaire)

"We must cultivate our own garden.
When man was put in the garden of Eden
he was put there so that he should work,
which proves that man was not born to rest."
- François-Marie Arouet (aka Voltaire)

"I love, live, and breath yoga, teaching people yoga.
It's the greatest sense of self care you can give yourself.
I love the energy connection with others
and seeing their transformations."
- Michelle Atwater

"Running is one the best solutions to a clear mind."
- Sasha Azevedo

"Happiness isn't in the future, it's not somewhere else.
It's available right inside us, right now, all the time."
- Leo Babauta

"On the topic of exercise,
It's just as important as brushing your teeth everyday,
more important than watching TV
or reading online or answering email.
Make time for something so crucial to a good life."
- Leo Babauta

"Principle 1: By setting limitations, we must choose the essential.
So in everything you do, learn to set limitations.
Principle 2: By choosing the essential, we create great impact
with minimal resources. Always choose the essential to
maximize your time and energy."
- Leo Babauta

"The life you have left is a gift. Cherish it.
Enjoy it now, to the fullest. Do what matters, now."
- Leo Babauta

"A healthy body is a guest-chamber for the soul;
a sick body is a prison."
- Francis Bacon

"I will never be an old man.
To me, old age is always 15 years older than I am."
- Francis Bacon

"Nature, to be commanded, must be obeyed."
- Francis Bacon

"I'm a vegetarian - I think there's a strong possibility,
had I not become a vegetarian, I would not be working now.
I became a vegetarian about 25 years ago,
and I did it out of concern for animals.
But I immediately began having more energy
and feeling better."
- Bob Barker

"I think that age as a number is not nearly as important as health.
You can be in poor health and be pretty miserable at 40 or 50.
If you're in good health, you can enjoy things into your 80s."
- Bob Barker

"The foundation of success in life is good health:
that is the substratum fortune;
it is also the basis of happiness.
A person cannot accumulate a fortune
very well when he is sick."
- P. T. Barnum

"As far away as you can get from the process
of mechanisms and machinery,
the more likely your food's going to taste good.
And that - that is probably the largest thing I can hand to
Anybody is let your hands touch it. Let them make it."
- Mario Batali

"I put hibiscus flower in every cup of tea I have.
It's sweet, sexy, and cleansing."
- Mario Batali

"Just because you eat doesn't mean you eat smart.
It's hard to beat a $1.99 wing pack of three at a fast-food restaurant
- it's so cheap - but that wing pack isn't feeding anyone,
it's just pushing hunger back an hour."
- Mario Batali

"Protein has been intensely over-represented on the plate.
Now, the garden should be the main drag for main courses."
- Mario Batali

"The kitchen really is the castle itself.
This is where we spend our happiest moments
and where we find the joy of being a family."
- Mario Batali

"When you cut that eggplant up and you roast it in the oven
and you make the tomato sauce and you put it on top,
your soul is in that food, and there's something about that
that can never be made by a company that
has three million employees."
- Mario Batali

"The body is like a piano, and happiness is like music.
It is needful to have the instrument in good order."
- Henry Ward Beecher

"Creating ways to be happy is your life's work,
a challenge that won't end until you die."
- Martha Beck

"Fact: From quitting smoking to skiing,
we succeed to the degree we try, fail, and learn.
Studies show that people who worry about mistakes shut down,
but those who are relaxed about doing badly soon learn to do well.
Success is built on failure."
- Martha Beck

"If something feels really good for you, you might want to do it.
And if it feels really horrible,
you might want to consider not doing it."
- Martha Beck

"People are so afraid of authority figures
and doctors are authority figures."
- Martha Beck

"Rest until you feel like playing,
then play until you feel like resting, period.
Never do anything else."
- Martha Beck

"I'm a very, very healthy eater. I eat lots of fish,
lots of vegetables, lots of fruit. I don't eat junk food."
- Victoria Beckham

"Eat real food, poop real often, feel real good.
It's that simple."
- Kathy Bee

"If it's white, don't bite.
It's best to stay away from refined, processed foods".
- Kathy Bee

"Drink only non-calorie containing beverages,
the best choices being water and green tea."
- John Berardi

"Eat every 2 - 3 hours, no matter what.
You should eat between 5 - 8 meals per day."
- John Berardi

"Health and fitness is your birthright."
- John Berardi

"My research focused primarily on exercise nutrition;
specifically, what to eat before, during
and after exercise to optimize performance."
- John Berardi

"Happiness is good health and a bad memory."
- Ingrid Bergman

"I was raised really, really healthy,
pretty much vegetarian and a very clean lifestyle,
I don't smoke, I don't drink. I'm more addicted to
the things that make me feel good
- endorphins after working out."
- Elizabeth Berkley

"Whenever you notice your thoughts detour into attack mode,
say out loud or to yourself:
'Happiness is a choice I make'."
- Gabrielle Bernstein

"There are lots of people in this world who spend so much time
watching their health that they haven't the time to enjoy it."
- Josh Billings

"Let me pose you a question.
Can farm-raised salmon be organic
when its feed has nothing to do with its natural diet,
even if the feed itself is supposedly organic, and the fish themselves
are packed tightly in pens, swimming in their own filth?"
- Mark Bittman

"This evidence is overwhelming at this point.
You eat more plants, you eat less other stuff, you live longer."
- Mark Bittman

"The USDA is not our ally here.
We have to take matters into our own hands,
not only by advocating for a better diet for everyone -
and that's the hard part - but by improving our own.
And that happens to be quite easy.
Less meat, less junk, more plants."
- Mark Bittman

"If I'd known I was going to live this long,
I'd have taken better care of myself."
- Eubie Blake

"Making my thoughts more positive
help me become stronger mentally,
which helps me push past any barrier,
be it physical or mental."
- Shaun "T" Blokker

"Want an excuse to do a surgery,
just do an MRI."
- Mike Boyle

"You never see anyone who can run or jump
who doesn't have an ass - in any sporting activity."
- Mike Boyle

"Fearlessly accept the reality; then fearlessly set
about transforming what needs to change."
- Elena Brower

"Yoga has led us not only to the beauty,
magic and majesty of our bodies,
but to the opportunities to make it right with ourselves,
and right with our families."
- Elena Brower

"Every human being is the author
of his own health or disease."
- Gautama Buddha

"Health is the greatest gift, contentment the greatest wealth,
faithfulness the best relationship."
- Gautama Buddha

"Holding on to anger is like grasping a hot coal with
the intent of throwing it at someone else;
you are the one who gets burned."
- Gautama Buddha

"Let us rise up and be thankful,
for if we didn't learn a lot at least we learned a little,
and if we didn't learn a little, at least we didn't get sick,
and if we got sick, at least we didn't die;
so, let us all be thankful."
- Gautama Buddha

"Peace comes from within. Do not seek it without."
- Gautama Buddha

"The secret of health for both mind and body
is not to mourn for the past,
not to worry about the future,
or not to anticipate troubles,
but to live the present moment wisely and earnestly."
- Gautama Buddha

"To enjoy good health,
to bring true happiness to one's family,
to bring peace to all, one must first discipline
and control one's own mind.
If a man can control his mind he can find
the way to Enlightenment,
and all wisdom and virtue will naturally come to him."
- Gautama Buddha

"To keep the body in good health is a duty,
otherwise we shall not be able to
keep our mind strong and clear."
- Gautama Buddha

"It's really up to us as individuals
to take control of our lives
and how we view our bodies.
Some of us are plump and curvy while others
are petite and can't put on weight.
There isn't a 'better' body or ideal type.
The sooner we can understand that,
the sooner we can get on and enjoy our lives
instead of how we think we look in it."
- Kathryn Budig

"Nothing in excess is good for us,
so I always make sure
to balance my hard work with
recovery, rest, good food, and play."
- Kathryn Budig

"A long healthy life is no accident.
It begins with good genes,
but it also depends on good habits."
- Dan Buettner

"Black beans and soy beans are the cornerstones
of longevity diets around the world."
- Dan Buettner

"Centenarians are still living near their children
and feel loved and the expectation to love.
Instead of being mere recipients of care,
they are contributors to the lives of their families.
They grow gardens to contribute vegetables,
they continue to cook and clean."
- Dan Buettner

"Clean water is the best longevity beverage on earth.
The Adventists believe you should drink seven glasses a day
- which can keep your arteries flowing better
and organs functioning higher.
We also found that herbal and green teas
probably have a strong longevity claim."
- Dan Buettner

"Exercise, from a public health perspective, is an unmitigated failure.
The world's longest-lived people live in environments
that nudge them into more movement.
They don't use power tools, they do their own yard work,
they grow a garden."
- Dan Buettner

"Food is the entrance ramp for better living."
- Dan Buettner

"Have fun, be active.
Ride a bike instead of driving, for example."
- Dan Buettner

"Having a purpose and knowing exactly what your values are
will add additional years to your life."
- Dan Buettner

"I can tell you that the longest-lived are getting 95%
of their calories from plants and only 5% from animal products.
Contrary to what the Paleo or Atkins diet says,
these folks actually eat a high carb diet.
About 65% of their diet is whole grains, beans and starchy tubers.
No matter where you go, the snack of choice is nuts.
People who eat nuts live 2-3 years longer than non-nut eaters."
- Dan Buettner

"Inconvenience yourself: ditch the remote, the garage door opener,
the leaf-blower; buy a bike, broom, rake, and snow shovel."
- Dan Buettner

"I think we live in a culture that relentlessly pursues comfort.
Ease is related to disease. We shouldn't always be fleeing hardship.
Hardship also brings people together.
We should welcome it."
- Dan Buettner

"One of the big things I've learned is that there's
an advantage to regular low-intensity activity."
- Dan Buettner

"The longest-lived people eat a plant-based diet.
They eat meat but only as a condiment or a celebration.
Nothing they eat has a plastic wrapper."
- Dan Buettner

"The people you surround yourself with influence your behaviors,
so choose friends who have healthy habits."
- Dan Buettner

"Walking is the only way proven to stave off
cognitive decline - it works."
- Dan Buettner

"Flowers always make people better, happier, and more helpful;
they are sunshine, food and medicine for the soul."
- Luther Burbank

"If exercise could be packaged into a pill, it would be the
single most prescribed and beneficial medicine in the nation."
- Robert Butler

"Americans love to hear good things about their bad habits."
- T. Colin Campbell

"At this point, any scientist, doctor, journalist,
or policy maker who denies or minimizes the importance
of a whole food, plant-based diet for individual
and societal well-being simply isn't looking clearly at the facts.
There's just too much good evidence to ignore anymore."
- T. Colin Campbell

"Casein, and very likely all animal proteins,
may be the most relevant
cancer-causing substances that we consume."
- T. Colin Campbell

"Costs have so consistently outpaced inflation that
we now spend one out of every seven dollars
the economy produces on health care."
- T. Colin Campbell

"Every kilogram of beef requires 100,000 liters of water to produce.
By comparison, a kilogram of wheat requires just 900 liters,
and a kilogram of potatoes just 500 liters."
- T. Colin Campbell

"Everything in food works together to create health or disease.
The more we think that a single chemical characterizes a whole
food, the more we stray into idiocy."
- T. Colin Campbell

"Fact is that certain people are making an awful lot of money today
selling foods that are unhealthy.
They want you to keep eating the foods they sell,
even though doing so makes you fat,
depletes your vitality and shortens and degrades your life.
They want you docile, compliant and ignorant."
- T. Colin Campbell

"Good health is about being able to fully enjoy the time we do have.
It is about being as functional as possible throughout our entire lives
and avoiding crippling, painful and lengthy battles with disease.
There are many better ways to die, and to live."
- T. Colin Campbell

"I have heard one doctor call high-protein, high-fat, low-
carbohydrate diets 'make-yourself-sick' diets,
and I think that's an appropriate moniker.
You can also lose weight by undergoing chemotherapy
or starting a heroin addiction,
but I wouldn't recommend those, either."
- T. Colin Campbell

"In one study of ten countries,
a higher consumption of calcium
was associated with a higher
- not lower risk of bone fracture."
- T. Colin Campbell

"It's never too late to start eating well.
A good diet can reverse many of those conditions as well.
In short: change the way you eat and
you can transform your health for the better."
- T. Colin Campbell

"Nutrients from animal-based foods
increased tumor development while nutrients from
plant-based foods decreased tumor development."
- T. Colin Campbell

"Other countries spend, on average, only about one-half
of what the U.S. spends per capita on health care.
Isn't it reasonable, therefore, for us to expect
our system to rank above theirs?
Unfortunately, among these twelve countries,
the U.S. system is consistently among the worst performers."
- T. Colin Campbell

"Population studies begun forty to fifty years ago show that
when people migrate from one country to another,
they acquire the cancer rate of the country to which they move,
despite the fact their genes remain the same."
- T. Colin Campbell

"Side effects of those very same prescription drugs
are the third leading cause of death,
behind heart disease and cancer. That's right!
Prescription drugs kill more people
than traffic accidents. According to Dr. Barbara Starfield,
writing in the Journal of the American Medical Association in 2000,
'adverse effects of medications'
(from drugs that were correctly prescribed and taken)
kill 106,000 people per year.
And that doesn't include accidental overdoses."
- T. Colin Campbell

"So how does the plant manage these complex reactions
and protect against errant electrons and free radicals?
It puts up a shield around potentially dangerous reactions
that sponges up these highly reactive substances.
The shield is made up of antioxidants
that intercept and scavenge electrons
that might otherwise stray from their course."
- T. Colin Campbell

"The foods you consume can heal you faster and
more profoundly than the most expensive prescription drugs,
and more dramatically than the
most extreme surgical interventions,
with only positive side effects."
- T. Colin Campbell

"These days, the supplement industry has the process down
to a 'science'. New scientific research on single nutrients
generalizes in a very superficial way about their ability
to promote human health. Companies put these newly
discovered 'nutrients' into pills, organize
public relations campaigns, and write marketing plans
to encourage a confused public to buy."
- T. Colin Campbell

"Wait until you're really sick',
could be the motto of doctors and hospitals in the current system.
'We can do nothing for you until your symptoms surpass the
subclinical and reveal themselves in pain, loss of function,
or a particularly worrisome test result.
Until then, keep calm and keep
eating the Standard American Diet'."
- T. Colin Campbell

"What made this project especially remarkable is that,
among the many associations that are relevant to diet and disease,
so many pointed to the same finding: people who ate the most
animal-based foods got the most chronic disease.
Even relatively small intakes of animal-based food were associated
with adverse effects. People who ate the most plant-based foods
were the healthiest and tended to avoid chronic disease."
- T. Colin Campbell

"You can't patent a recommendation to eat lots of fruits,
vegetables, nuts, seeds, and whole grains.
So there's no incentive for industry to invest in such research
and no incentive for researchers to study and validate such claims."
- T. Colin Campbell

"Exercise is the main thing that helped me lose weight."
- Drew Carey

"I always run in the morning on an empty stomach,
and I'll go through a bottle and a half of water.
Then I have a protein drink or I eat egg whites."
- Drew Carey

"I always thought I was going to die before I was 60."
- Drew Carey

"I am never out there just jogging for the heck of it.
I never do that. I start to run with a goal in mind,
whether it's a certain time or certain distance or
a specific heart-rate goal, and then I am done."
- Drew Carey

"I was just sick of being fat, you know?
You get sick of it. It just really, it's a tiring lifestyle to have."
- Drew Carey

"The easiest diet is, you know, eat vegetables, eat fresh food.
Just a really sensible healthy diet like you read about all the time."
- Drew Carey

"The hardest diet I was ever on was the one when I was fat.
You can only wear fat clothes, you don't feel good,
your sex life gets damaged,
you don't have energy for anything. It's horrible."
- Drew Carey

"I think I have to remain eternally oblivious to age.
Honestly, when you put a number on it yourself,
it's just like, Why? Why do that?"
- Mariah Carey

"Since having the babies, I realize that 90 percent
of losing weight is my diet."
- Mariah Carey

"He who has health, has hope,
and he who has hope, has everything."
- Thomas Carlyle

"Change your plate. Change your fate."
- Kris Carr

"If you don't think your anxiety, depression, sadness
and stress impact your physical health, think again.
All of these emotions trigger
chemical reactions in your body,
which can lead to inflammation
and a weakened immune system.
Learn how to cope, sweet friend.
There will always be dark days."
- Kris Carr

"If you really want to turn your health around,
start juicing today."
- Kris Carr

"I knew when I was diagnosed with cancer
the only thing I could control was what I ate,
what I drank and what I would think."
- Kris Carr

"Processed foods cause inflammation,
a source of most chronic illnesses as well as stress."
- Kris Carr

"There's a great metaphor that one of my doctors uses:
If a fish is swimming in a dirty tank and it gets sick,
do you take it to the vet and amputate the fin?
No, you clean the water. So, I cleaned up my system.
By eating organic raw greens, nuts and healthy fats,
I am flooding my body with enzymes, vitamins and oxygen."
- Kris Carr

"Whether you're reaching for one of your favorite cookbooks
or just winging it, do your best to keep a well-stocked arsenal
of healthy ingredients at your disposal.
At the very least, you'll always be ready to
whip up a green juice or smoothie.
- Kris Carr

"The mind controls so much of the body.
We are much more than flesh and blood;
we are complex systems.
Patients do better when they have faith
that they're going to do better.
That's why I always tell my patients and their families
not to neglect their prayers.
There's nobody I don't say that to."
- Ben Carson

"We should be concerned not only about
the health of individual patients,
but also the health of our entire society."
- Ben Carson

"Education can help all Americans live longer, healthier lives.
Teaching students to make healthy decisions
can improve habits now and instill
healthy eating habits for a lifetime."
- Matt Cartwright

"Nutrition isn't the only problem;
our children also aren't getting enough exercise."
- Matt Cartwright

"Unhealthy eating habits cause major health problems,
such as diabetes and heart disease,
and can also lead to food insecurity,
disrupted eating patterns, and low self-esteem."
- Matt Cartwright

"Animals that we eat are raised for food
in the most economical way possible,
and the serious food producers do it
in the most humane way possible.
I think anyone who is a carnivore
needs to understand
that meat does not originally come
in these neat little packages."
- Julia Child

"As we say in the American Institute of Wine and Food,
small helpings, no seconds. A little bit of everything.
No snacking. And have a good time."
- Julia Child

"The perfect dressing is essential to the perfect salad,
and I see no reason whatsoever for using a bottled dressing,
which may have been sitting on the grocery shelf
for weeks, even months - even years."
- Julia Child

"Don't put off living to next week, next month,
next year or next decade.
The only time you're ever living is in this moment."
- Celestine Chua

"If insurance companies paid for lifestyle-management classes,
they would save huge sums of money. We need to see
that alternative medicine is now mainstream."
- Deepak Chopra

"If we are creating ourselves all the time,
then it is never too late to begin creating the bodies we want
instead of the ones we mistakenly assume we are stuck with."
- Deepak Chopra

"I, of course, meditate for two hours every morning.
It's part of my schedule;
I wake up at 4 am every day and I love it."
- Deepak Chopra

"Modern medicine, for all its advances,
knows less than 10 percent of what your body knows instinctively."
- Deepak Chopra

"Preventive medicine isn't part of a physician's everyday routine,
which is spent dispensing drugs and performing surgery."
- Deepak Chopra

"The real secret to lifelong good health is actually the opposite:
Let your body take care of you."
- Deepak Chopra

"The way you think, the way you behave, the way you eat,
can influence your life by 30 to 50 years."
- Deepak Chopra

"Adopting a new healthier lifestyle can involve changing diet
to include more fresh fruit and vegetables
as well as increasing levels of exercise."
- Linford Christie

"Healthy citizens are the greatest asset
any country can have."
- Winston S. Churchill

"Always keep it simple!
Even after increasing your habit, all repetitions must remain easy.
The total habit should be broken down into easier pieces if needed."
- James Clear

"Don't push happiness off until you hit some future milestone.
Allow yourself to be happy in the moment.
Be happy while you are working on the task.
While you are working on building your skill set,
rather than thinking it is something you will get to
once you are good enough."
- James Clear

"Focus on what you really want to achieve
and remove all surrounding distractions."
- James Clear

"Generate a system. Plan out how you will stick to your habits,
how are you going to stay passionate and focused?"
- James Clear

"If you're considering a new diet,
but you're worried that you might not be able to stick with it
when you go out with your friends on Thursday nights,
then you're worrying about an edge case.
Thursday night isn't going to make or break you.
It's the work you put in during the other twenty meals
of the week that matters."
- James Clear

"If you want to eat more vegetables,
you could limit yourself to only one type of vegetable this week.
By limiting the number of choices you have to make,
it's more likely that you'll actually eat something healthy
rather than get overwhelmed trying to figure out
all of the details of the perfect diet."
- James Clear

"If you want to start exercising, set a rule for yourself where
you are not allowed to exercise for more than five minutes.
You have to stop exercising after five minutes.
I talked with a reader named Mitch
who used this strategy to make
his first six weeks of exercise very easy and
then gradually built up to doing more.
He ended up losing over 100 pounds."
- James Clear

"My work is focused on a simple idea:
I want to share practical ideas and proven research
that helps you master your habits, optimize your performance,
and take control of your health and happiness."
- James Clear

"You have to start with a version of the habit
that is incredibly easy for you.
It must be so easy that you can't say no to doing it
and so easy that it is not difficult at all in the beginning."
- James Clear

"You have to increase your habit each day,
but in an incredibly small way."
- James Clear

"Any family doctor will tell you that people will stay healthier
and long-term of cost to the health system will be lower
if we have comprehensive preventive services.
You know how all of our mothers told us that an ounce
of prevention was worth a pound of cure?
Our mothers were right."
- Bill Clinton

"Despite the dedication of literally millions
of talented health care professionals,
our health care is too uncertain and too expensive,
too bureaucratic and too wasteful.
It has too much fraud and too much greed."
- Bill Clinton

"Drug companies should no longer charge
three times more for prescription drugs
made in America here in the United States
than they charge for the same drugs overseas."
- Bill Clinton

"In recent years the number of administrators in our hospitals
has grown by four times the rate
that the number of doctors has grown.
A hospital ought to be a house of healing,
not a monument to paperwork and bureaucracy."
- Bill Clinton

"Our medical bills are growing at over twice the rate of inflation,
and the United States spends over a third more
of its income on health care than any other nation on earth."
- Bill Clinton

"Running helps me stay on an even keel
and in an optimistic frame of mind."
- Bill Clinton

"School is where children spend most of their time,
and it is where we lay the foundation for healthy habits.
That's why New Jersey is the first state to adopt
a comprehensive school nutrition policy
that bans candy, soda, and other junk food."
- Richard J. Codey

"Walking is magic. Can't recommend it highly enough.
I read that Plato and Aristotle did much of their
brilliant thinking together while ambulating.
The movement, the meditation, the health of the blood pumping,
and the rhythm of footsteps... this is a primal way
to connect with one's deeper self."
- Paula Cole

"I don't know too many parents
that want to feed their kids soda,
but high-fructose corn syrup is cheap.
The price of soda in 20 years has gone down 40 percent
while the price of whole foods, fruits and vegetables,
has gone up 40 percent
and obesity goes up right along that curve."
- Tom Colicchio

"Remember, the feeling you get from a good run is far better
than the feeling you get from sitting around
wishing you were running."
- Sarah Condor

"Don't put all your health and fitness eggs in one basket.
Work equally hard on your nutrition, exercise,
cognitive skills, and personality."
- Bret Contreras

"If you think lifting weights is dangerous, try being weak.
Being weak is dangerous."
- Bret Contreras

"Being strong doesn't mean much
without fluid, efficient movement."
- Gray Cook

"First move well, then move often."
- Gray Cook

"1. If you can't test it, don't train it
2. Go light and do it right
3. Balance is the base."
- Gray Cook

"If you want to see your abs eat better.
If you want your abs to work better, move better!"
- Gray Cook

"Moving isn't important, until you can't."
- Gray Cook

"Original humans were on their feet
for a large part of the day without leisure
or entertainment opportunities
designed around sitting in one place."
- Gray Cook

"Pain is not the problem - it's the signal."
- Gray Cook

"Quitting unproductive practices early and
moving on to something better
is a hallmark of successful people."
- Gray Cook

"Some of the fittest people in the world don't obsess
about their exercise time slot -
they don't require loud music or mirrors to motivate them.
They simply practice movement skills,
knowing they will never master them.
They use exercise correctly and
they stay in touch with movement.
Exercise correctness is not a popular topic,
but is a much needed perspective."
- Gray Cook

"Tarzan, to me, is the epitome of fitness.
The guy is strong, agile and quick.
He can run, jump, climb and swing through trees.
If we take a person who moves well and put them on a
Crossfit type of training program, we turn them into Tarzan.
If we take that same program and give it to the majority
of people in society who move poorly,
we turn them into a patient."
- Gray Cook

"The definition of functional exercise is what it produces,
NOT what it looks like."
- Gray Cook

"The number one risk factor for musculoskeletal injury
is a previous injury, implying that our rehabilitation process
is missing something."
- Gray Cook

"The only thing documented for depression
that does not have side effects is exercise."
- Gray Cook

"When someone's back hurts they don't want to blame
their lifestyle, fitness level, or daily patterns.
Instead, they want to blame their back pain
on starting the lawn mower last week, which in reality,
is probably just the straw that broke the camel's back.
Human beings live under the philosophy of,
'I have a snowball and I have to throw it at someone'.
No one wants to take responsibility."
- Gray Cook

"While some serious injuries are unavoidable
and need surgical repair,
we should do everything possible to build an
injury buffer zone by training healthy movement.
It is always better to bend than break -
and strong agile bodies bend better than weak, stiff bodies."
- Gray Cook

"You gotta break a pattern before you can make a pattern!"
- Gray Cook

"I don't criticize weight training -
as long as it is not a substitute for aerobic training."
- Kenneth H. Cooper

"I have not missed a day from work because of illness since 1956."
- Kenneth H. Cooper

"The reason I exercise is for the quality of life I enjoy."
- Kenneth H. Cooper

"We are involved in youth testing internationally.
We want to try to prove without a shadow of a doubt
the relationship between physical fitness and health,
not just physical fitness and ability to perform."
- Kenneth H. Cooper

"Chronic malnutrition, or the lack of proper nutrition
over time directly contributes to three times
as many child deaths as food scarcity.
Yet surprisingly, you don't really hear about this
hidden crisis through the morning news,
Twitter or headlines of major newspapers."
- Cat Cora

"I believe that parents need to make nutrition education
a priority in their home environment.
It's crucial for good health and longevity to instill
in your children sound eating habits from an early age."
- Cat Cora

"Research shows that what works and is healthy for adults
also works well for children, if adjusted to be age-appropriate.
Children, like adults, do not suffer from a deficiency
of white sugar, white flour, junk food, or processed foods.
A growing child as well as an adult is hurt by
junk foods and benefited by healthy foods."
- Gabriel Cousens

"Hearty laughter is a good way to jog internally
without having to go outdoors."
- Norman Cousins

"It is reasonable to expect the doctor to recognize
that science may not have all the answers to
problems of health and healing."
- Norman Cousins

"The capacity for hope is the most significant fact of life.
It provides human beings with a sense of destination
and the energy to get started."
- Norman Cousins

"The human body experiences a powerful
gravitational pull in the direction of hope.
That is why the patient's hopes
are the physician's secret weapon.
They are the hidden ingredients in any prescription."
- Norman Cousins

"Your heaviest artillery will be your will to live.
Keep that big gun going."
- Norman Cousins

"More than ever,
you need to be an advocate for your health."
- Eric Cressey

"Happiness lies, first of all, in health."
- George William Curtis

"Be gone excuses."
- Chantal Dalabona

"Growing up, my mother always told me to
eat my vegetables so I could have dessert,
even though my taste buds didn't like it one bit.
Exercising can be a bit like eating vegetables.
You whine, you pull faces, maybe even break a sweat,
but oh, that sweet reward in the end makes it all worthwhile."
- Chantal Dalabona

"Keep it simple. It's the little things you do everyday that make
a world of difference in your health & overall state of being."
- Chantal Dalabona

"Physical fitness is a gift we give to ourselves that allows us
to innately discover our immense capacity to thrive."
- Chantal Dalabona

"When you accept the invitation to embrace a healthier lifestyle,
a transformational shift happens.
You have just given yourself permission to
gain energy, clarity and strength by doing the things
you need to do and trusting in the process."
- Chantal Dalabona

"Your body is a beautiful gift,
the only one you have,
so how about giving it some loving."
- Chantal Dalabona

"Balance is strength."
- Marco Dalabona

"I've never met anyone who has
started lifting and gotten weaker."
- Marco Dalabona

"Running long and hard is an ideal antidepressant,
since it's hard to run and
feel sorry for yourself at the same time."
- Monte Davis

"Any doctor will admit... you see if you're put
on high blood pressure drugs,
they'll tell you that you'll be on them the rest of your life.
Why? Because they don't cure anything,
They only cover up the symptoms."
- Lorraine Day

"After discovering cancer,
I changed my diet completely."
- Lorraine Day

"Caffeine is an abnormal stimulant."
- Lorraine Day

"Cancer doesn't scare me anymore."
- Lorraine Day

"Diseases just don't happen."
- Lorraine Day

"Drugs and surgery is all we were taught in medical school."
- Lorraine Day

"If people go on a vegetarian diet,
exercise on a regular basis and decrease alcohol intake,
a study done at Harvard School of Public Health
revealed that they will decrease the incidence of cancer by 66%."
- Lorraine Day

"In medical journal articles that doctors read,
there are more pages in the medical journal of 4-color
high priced pharmaceutical ads,
then there is medical information!"
- Lorraine Day

"The body is made to heal itself."
- Lorraine Day

"We give these diseases to ourselves one day at a time
by what we eat and the way we live."
- Lorraine Day

"What we're eating is actually destroying us.
It's actually causing cancer and other diseases."
- Lorraine Day

"You cannot develop cancer unless your
immune system is suppressed."
- Lorraine Day

"We don't have to get sick as we get older."
- Aubrey de Grey

"When you look at people around the world who live past 100,
the one thing they all share in common
is a laid back happy attitude."
- Aubrey de Grey

"I really believe the only way to stay healthy is to eat properly,
get your rest and exercise.
If you don't exercise and do the other two,
I still don't think it's going to help you that much."
- Mike Ditka

"The power of love to change bodies is legendary,
built into folklore, common sense, and everyday experience.
Love moves the flesh, it pushes matter around.
Throughout history, 'tender loving care' has uniformly
been recognized as a valuable element in healing."
- Larry Dossey

"For the first 50 years of your life
the food industry is trying to make you fat.
Then, the second 50 years,
the pharmaceutical industry is treating you for everything."
- Pierre Dukan

"I go jogging for 25 minutes every morning,
even if I'm away from home."
- Pierre Dukan

"It's been proven that fitting more activity
into your day can greatly improve your health."
- Pierre Dukan

"If you put on weight it's not by chance.
You put on weight because you eat compulsively."
- Pierre Dukan

"There is nothing unhealthy about
educating youngsters about nutrition."
- Pierre Dukan

"To be a nutritionist in France,
you must be a doctor, seven years studies,
and then three more years in nutrition."
- Pierre Dukan

"You never see a French person eating alone."
- Pierre Dukan

"Kids are killing themselves with energy drinks.
Literally, in my health seminars I show parents
the newspaper articles of all these teenagers who've died
from drinking too many energy drinks!"
- Scott duPont

"Great health is the KEY to every other part of your life."
- Scott duPont

"The old adage: 'Doing the same exact things every day and
expecting different results is the definition of insanity'.
This is especially true with your health.
The great news is a few small changes in your daily habits
and routines can lead to massive results!"
- Scott duPont

"For 99% of the people I work with, I tell them:
'There's NO excuse for not walking,
or at least moving every day'.
If it's below freezing outside, dress warm.
If you can't stand, use a walker.
If you have no legs, use your arms to push your wheelchair.
If you stop moving, you're dying!"
- Scott duPont

"I always try to buy 'locally grown, in season' food.
It's usually less expensive and
a lot better for you & our environment
than shipping produce 10,000 miles around the world
for your next meal."
- Scott duPont

"I encourage my clients to change how they
describe their fitness activities:
'Exercising & Energizing' sounds better
than 'Working Out'.
'Getting Pumped Up' sounds more appealing
than 'Lifting Heavy Weights'.
'Biking by the lake' seems like more fun than
'Gotta climb the stair master for 30 minutes'."
- Scott duPont

"More people need to realize how incredibly harmful
sugar is to all aspects of their health.
Just like the taxes now on tobacco products,
the best deterrent (and solution) will be
a tax on foods with ridiculously high sugar content."
- Scott duPont

"Pay attention and listen to your body after you eat different foods.
Over time you will find foods that give you more energy
and simply make you feel great!"
- Scott duPont

"People think I'm excessive making a priority of exercising
every single day including Sunday & Holidays, thinking I should rest.
My reasoning is exercise gives me lots of energy,
clears my head & I feel great!
Why wouldn't I want to have tons of energy
and feel great every day?"
- Scott duPont

"Unless you prioritize time EVERY DAY
for yourself & your health, things will never change.
Don't wait until tomorrow."
- Scott duPont

"My mother was a P.E. teacher,
and she was kind of a fanatic
about fitness and nutrition growing up,
so it was ingrained in me at a young age.
As I get older, I'm finding out it's not about getting
all buffed up and looking good.
It's more about staying healthy and flexible."
- Josh Duhamel

"Shifting to a low-sugar, lower carbohydrate diet
is particularly important for people looking to
lose weight or repair their metabolism,
and it seems prudent for everyone."
- John Durant

"There are serious environmental and ethical problems
with the industrial food system."
- John Durant

"A home gym is great,
but only if you have the motivation to use it.
Training in a home gym has to be scheduled
just like an appointment.
It's got to be part of your schedule and
become part of your lifestyle."
- Todd Durkin

"Permit yourself at least two weeks
of 'mellow yellow' time per year.
This is time on vacation. Vacation time and time away is critical
to restore and reenergize your spirit.
Book it in advance and don't change it!"
- Todd Durkin

"Set up your home gym so it's your sacred space.
Put up motivational quotes on the wall,
hang pictures that inspire you.
Put a few plants in there and let some natural sunlight in.
Make it a place you want to work out in,
a place where you want to go to take care of yourself."
- Todd Durkin

"Take care of YOU."
- Todd Durkin

"Be miserable. Or motivate yourself.
Whatever has to be done,
it's always your choice."
- Wayne Dyer

"Doing what you love is the cornerstone of
having abundance in your life."
- Wayne Dyer

"It is impossible for you to be angry and laugh at the same time.
Anger and laughter are mutually exclusive
and you have the power to choose either."
- Wayne Dyer

"It makes no sense to worry
about things you have no control over
because there's nothing you can do about them,
and why worry about things you do control?
The activity of worrying keeps you immobilized."
- Wayne Dyer

"Simply put, you believe that things
or people make you unhappy,
but this is not accurate.
You make yourself unhappy.
- Wayne Dyer

"Stop acting as if life is a rehearsal.
Live this day as if it were your last.
The past is over and gone.
The future is not guaranteed."
- Wayne Dyer

"There is no scarcity of opportunity to
make a living at what you love;
there's only scarcity of resolve to make it happen."
- Wayne Dyer

"When you dance, your purpose is not to get to
a certain place on the floor.
It's to enjoy each step along the way."
- Wayne Dyer

"When you judge another, you do not define them,
you define yourself."
- Wayne Dyer

"You cannot be lonely if
you like the person you're alone with."
- Wayne Dyer

"The doctor of the future will give no medicines,
but will interest his patients in the care of the human frame,
in diet, and in the causes and prevention of disease."
- Thomas Edison

"Life is like riding a bicycle.
To keep your balance, you must keep moving."
- Albert Einstein

"Nothing happens until something starts moving."
- Albert Einstein

"People need to realize that there's no such thing as a
'Lipitor deficiency' or a 'Crestor deficiency',
yet we keep taking these types of pills every day."
- Bruce Ellington

"Prevention is better than cure."
- Desiderius Erasmus

"Cholesterol is a white, waxy substance that
is not found in plants - only in animals.
It is an essential component of the membrane that
coats all our cells, and it is the basic ingredient of sex hormones.
Our bodies need cholesterol,
and they manufacture it on their own. We do not need to eat it.
But we do, when we consume meat, poultry, fish, and
other animal-based foods, such as dairy products and eggs.
In doing so, we take on excess amounts of the substance.
What's more, eating fat (even as added oil) causes the body
itself to manufacture excessive amounts of cholesterol,
which explains why vegetarians who eat oil, butter, cheese, milk,
ice cream, glazed doughnuts, and French pastry
develop coronary disease despite their avoidance of meat."
- Caldwell Esselstyn

"Collectively, the media; the meat, oil, and dairy industries;
most prominent chefs and cookbook authors; and our own
government are not presenting accurate advice
about the healthiest way to eat."
- Caldwell Esselstyn

"Every mouthful of oils and animal products, including dairy foods,
initiates an assault on these (cell) membranes and,
therefore, on the cells they protect.
These foods produce a cascade of free radicals in our bodies -
especially harmful chemical substances that induce metabolic
injuries from which there is only a partial recovery.
Year after year, the effects accumulate.
And eventually, the cumulative cell injury is
great enough to become obvious,
to express itself as what physicians define as disease.
Plants and grains do not induce the deadly cascade of free radicals.
Even better, in fact, they carry an antidote.
Unlike oils and animal products,
they contain antioxidants, which help to neutralize the
free radicals and also, recent research suggests, may provide
considerable protection against cancers."
- Caldwell Esselstyn

"I believe that coronary artery disease is preventable,
and that even after it is underway,
its progress can be stopped, its insidious effects reversed.
I believe, and my work over the past twenty years has
demonstrated, that all this can be accomplished without expensive
mechanical intervention and with minimal use of drugs.
The key lies in nutrition - specifically, in abandoning the toxic
American diet and maintaining cholesterol levels well below
those historically recommended by health policy experts."
- Caldwell Esselstyn

"The cost of this epidemic is enormous - greater,
by far, than that of any other disease.
The United States spends more than $250 billion
a year on heart disease.
But here is the truly shocking statistic:
nearly all that money is devoted to treating symptoms.
It pays for cardiac drugs, for clot-dissolving medications,
and for costly mechanical techniques that bypass clogged arteries
or widen them with balloons, tiny rotating knives, lasers, and stents.
All of these approaches carry significant risk of serious
complications, including death."
- Caldwell Esselstyn

"We should be aiming much higher:
at arresting coronary artery disease altogether,
even reversing its course. And the key to doing this,
as my research demonstrates, is not simply reducing the amount
of fat and cholesterol you ingest, but eliminating cholesterol
and any fat beyond the natural, healthy amounts
found in plants, from your diet.
The key is plant-based nutrition."
- Caldwell Esselstyn

"The doctor of the future will no longer treat the human frame
with drugs, but rather will cure and prevent disease with nutrition."
- Thomas Edison

"Nothing will benefit human health and increase the
chances for survival of life on earth as much as
the evolution to a vegetarian diet."
- Albert Einstein

"All the pre-made sauces in a jar, and frozen and canned
vegetables, processed meats, and cheeses which are
loaded with artificial ingredients and sodium
can get in the way of a healthy diet.
My number one advice is to eat fresh, and seasonally."
- Todd English

"First say to yourself what you would be;
and then do what you have to do."
- Epictetus

"It takes more than just a good looking body.
You've got to have the heart and soul to go with it."
- Epictetus

"Preach not to others what they should eat,
but eat as becomes you, and be silent."
- Epictetus

"The key is to keep company only with people who uplift you,
whose presence calls forth your best."
- Epictetus

"Most people focus on working OUT to lose weight,
but if you want to see results that
last a lifetime start working IN...
Change the Mind
Change the Body."
- Vanessa Esperanza

"We tend to look in the mirror and
focus on what we don't like...
If we just focus on what we do like,
we'll see more of THAT
next time we look in the mirror."
- Vanessa Esperanza

"Breathe, Relax, Let Go and Allow your Life to Flow."
- Sharon Feanny

"If you want to Detox it takes 3 days to Let Go,
7 Days to Renew and
21 Days to a Whole New You!"
- Sharon Feanny

"It's not just what you put in your body,
it's also what you put ON your body that matters!"
- Sharon Feanny

"My Mantra for a healthy and happy life is
Live Fit, Live Life and
Most Importantly, Live LOVE!"
- Sharon Feanny

"Stop counting calories in your food
and start counting the vitality that
the food you are eating will give you
- that's how you lose weight!"
- Sharon Feanny

"Take the peace that you found from
your yoga mat, into your world, share it with
everyone you encounter, and please,
use peace for every decision you have to make."
- Sharon Feanny

"Everyone is going to binge on a diet, for instance,
so plan for it, schedule it, and contain the damage."
- Tim Ferriss

"The first thing I would do for anyone who's trying to lose body fat,
for instance, would be to remove foods from the house
that he or she would consume during lapses of self-control."
- Tim Ferriss

"There is often an important difference between those
who succeed and those who fail: their levels of energy.
Every action we take requires a minimum amount of energy,
especially mental or psychic energy."
- Mark Fisher

"Go vegetable heavy.
Reverse the psychology of your plate
by making meat the side dish
and vegetables the main course."
- Bobby Flay

"Anyone can train hard.
Do you have the discipline to recover?"
- Lauren Fleshman

"I learned a long time ago that the last thing any woman
should be thinking about is being 'skinny' or 'thin.'
To me, those words imply weakness, fragility,
the inability to stand firm in a storm.
If you want to change your body, aim for 'athletic'.
An athletic body is healthy, strong, and built to thrive.
An athletic body can take many shapes."
- Lauren Fleshman

"I may not be the lithest, the most talented,
or have the fastest time in the field,
but I have passion and courage,
and sometimes that is enough
to do something extraordinary."
- Lauren Fleshman

"Make your race a playground,
not a proving ground."
- Lauren Fleshman

"Elsewhere the paper notes that vegetarians and vegans
(including athletes) 'meet and exceed requirements' for protein.
And, to render the whole
we-should-worry-about-getting-enough-protein
and therefore-eat-meat idea even more useless,
other data suggests that excess animal protein intake is linked
with osteoporosis, kidney disease, calcium stones
in the urinary tract, and some cancers.
Despite some persistent confusion,
it is clear that vegetarians and vegans
tend to have more optimal protein consumption than omnivores."
- Jonathan Safran Foer

"That's the Lean & Lovely intention -
to change your body by changing the way
you view and treat yourself."
- Neghar Fonooni

"Early to bed and early to rise makes a man
healthy, wealthy and wise."
- Benjamin Franklin

"Energy and persistence conquer all things."
- Benjamin Franklin

"Some people die at 25 and aren't buried until 75."
- Benjamin Franklin

"While we may not be able to control all that happens to us,
we can control what happens inside us."
- Benjamin Franklin

"I don't believe in diets."
- Bethenny Frankel

"Never eat while doing something else,
because you won't get
the satisfaction from your food
and you'll be more likely to overeat."
- Bethenny Frankel

"Your diet is a bank account.
Good food choices are good investments."
- Bethenny Frankel

"Changing my diet - first to vegetarian and then later to vegan
- made energy almost a non-issue for me.
I'm never tired until the very end of the day,
and that's very different from how I used to be,
even when I thought I ate pretty healthily."
- Matt Frazier

"I do so little 'consumption' (of TV, news, social media, blogs)
that I don't spend any energy at all on worrying
or thinking about current events."
- Matt Frazier

"There are many who don't understand
that it's possible to eat a healthy, substantial diet
that includes no animal products whatsoever."
- Matt Frazier

"If a box tries to convince you its contents are healthy,
there's a great chance that they're not."
- Yoni Freedhoff

"You shouldn't wish any days away.
You've got fewer than you think."
- Yoni Freedhoff

"Blueberries, strawberries and blackberries are true super foods.
Naturally sweet and juicy, berries are low in sugar
and high in nutrients -
they are among the best foods you can eat."
- Joel Fuhrman

"Eating a high-nutrient diet actually makes you
more satisfied with less food,
and actually gives the ability to
enjoy food more without overeating."
- Joel Fuhrman

"Food is really and truly the most effective medicine."
- Joel Fuhrman

"Healthy people eating healthy food
should never need to take an antibiotic."
- Joel Fuhrman

"In the future, it's going to become more and more impossible
for the economy to support how expensive medical care is
and the number of sick people we have.
Why don't we just get our population healthier
so we don't need medical care?"
- Joel Fuhrman

"Seeds and nuts are indispensable for cardiovascular health.
The protective properties of nuts against coronary heart disease
were first recognized in the early 1990s,
and a strong body of literature has followed,
confirming these original findings."
- Joel Fuhrman

"The modern diet is grossly deficient in hundreds of important plant-derived immunity-building compounds which makes us highly vulnerable to viruses, infections and disease."
- Joel Fuhrman

"To provide optimal levels of protective micronutrients, a diet must be vegetable-based, not grain-based."
- Joel Fuhrman

"We're not going to find a magic cure for cancer. We've got to prevent it."
- Joel Fuhrman

"The elements of water that make it good are a pH that's slightly alkaline and lots of electrons, because electrons are energy."
- Michael Galitzer

"It is health that is real wealth and not pieces of gold and silver."
- Mahatma Gandhi

"Don't let your values change with society; instead let your values change society."
- Tony A. Gaskins Jr.

"Let your pain birth your purpose. Let your mess become your message. Let this be a stepping-stone and not a stumbling block. Change."
- Tony A. Gaskins Jr.

"If you don't build your dream someone
will hire you to help build theirs."
- Tony A. Gaskins Jr.

"To be content doesn't mean you don't desire more,
it means you're thankful for what you have
and patience for what's to come."
- Tony Gaskins, Jr.

"Hunger, inadequate medical care, poor housing, and
inferior schools are enemies of the sense of wonder.
It is easier and less expensive in the long run to
prevent a loss of imagination by providing adequate nutrition,
housing, medical care, and schooling
than it is to try to restore that loss."
- Margaret Geller

"All chronic and degenerative diseases are caused
by two and only two major problems,
toxicity and deficiency."
- Charlotte Gerson

"For any ill individual as well as for someone
in a state of good health,
drinking fresh-made juices processed from
organically grown fruits and vegetables
frequently through each day is critical to
renewing or maintaining wellness."
- Charlotte Gerson

"Gabriel Feldman, M.D., director of the prostate
and colorectal cancer programs
for the American Cancer Society, admits,
'We don't need years of research.
If people would implement what we know today,
cancer rates would drop. It's that simple'.
Dr. Max Gerson was correct in his medical/nutritional
literary presentation of 1958
before the advent of fast food restaurants
and supermarket convenience foods,
and his intuitions are even more accurate today."
- Charlotte Gerson

"Is there a 'vital force' taken into the body from juice drinking?
It's strictly our opinion, but we say 'Yes!'
The live enzymes in vegetables and fruits may be absorbed
into the physical, mental, and spiritual self
and probably do invigorate one's soul."
- Charlotte Gerson

"It's safer to use foods in the most natural form,
combined and mixed by nature and raised,
if possible, by an organic gardening process,
thus obeying the laws of nature."
- Charlotte Gerson

"It's the doctors duty to activate and reactivate
the body's own healing mechanism."
- Charlotte Gerson

"Modern allopathic medicine is the only major science
stuck in the pre-Einstein era."
- Charlotte Gerson

"No attempt should be made to cure the body
without curing the soul',
wrote Plato nearly 2,400 years ago.
Body and mind are inseparable;
they sicken together and must be healed together."
- Charlotte Gerson

"When you change your diet,
you can change your entire physiology and you can heal."
- Charlotte Gerson

"You can't keep one disease and heal two others.
When the body heals, it heals everything."
- Charlotte Gerson

"You can't trash and pollute your body
and expect to have perfect health."
- Charlotte Gerson

"Stay close to nature and her eternal laws will protect you."
- Max Gerson

"Resist less, savor more...
Let yoga reframe your resilience regimen."
- DonnaLyn Giegerich

"Selfcare is the new healthcare.
Yoga helped save our lives!"
- DonnaLyn Giegerich

"Speak softly and carry a big yoga mat!"
- DonnaLyn Giegerich

"Want to lead and succeed?
Let yoga inform your leadership life!"
- DonnaLyn Giegerich

"Almost as soon as I went vegan,
people started telling me that my skin looked great,
and that I appeared younger, slimmer, and healthier.
I'm convinced that of all the changes I've made to my lifestyle,
it's the adoption of a vegan diet that has been best for me
- physically, mentally, and certainly spiritually."
- Stephen Glover (aka Steve-O)

"Cancer care will advance patient by patient.
As each cancer patient recovers his or her health,
thanks to alternative medicine, and tells a friend and
the family doctor, this will transform Western medicine."
- Burton Goldberg

"Doctors don't want to rock the boat.
They don't want to risk that the FDA will punish them
or their state medical board will yank away their license.
And I don't blame them."
- Burton Goldberg

"Have you ever had a conventional doctor
urge you to eat organic food?"
- Burton Goldberg

"I did this book 'Harvest for Hope,'
and I learned so much about food.
And one thing I learned is that we have the guts
not of a carnivore, but of an herbivore.
Herbivore guts are very long because they have
to get the last bit of nutrition out of leaves and things."
- Jane Goodall

"If you have health, you truly have everything."
- Janice Gordon

"Age is a question of mind over matter.
If you don't mind, it doesn't matter."
- Jon Gordon

"Decide right now the age you want to be."
- Jon Gordon

"I have found that the more often I live in the 'now',
the more energy I have.
Energy spent in the past or future is worthless now.
It's like investing money in a company
that already went bankrupt
or hasn't even been created yet."
- Jon Gordon

"It takes a lot more energy to keep positive energy
out of our lives than it does to let it in."
- Jon Gordon

"The energy we project is the energy we receive.
We are like a movie projector and what we project on
to the world's movie screen is what the world sees."
- Jon Gordon

"You stop moving, you're dead.
Then you're no fun."
- Brogan Graham

"Exercise is non negotiable,
an appointment you will not miss."
- Bob Greene

"We were made to exercise. We feel better."
- Bob Greene

"My own prescription for health is less paperwork
and more running barefoot through the grass."
- Leslie Grimutter

"By cleansing your body on a regular basis and eliminating
as many toxins as possible from your environment,
your body can begin to heal itself, prevent disease,
and become stronger and more resilient
than you ever dreamed possible!"
- Edward Group III

"Hate less, live longer."
- Terri Guillemets

"Health is a relationship between you and your body."
- Terri Guillemets

"Our bodies run on the fresh green fuel of the land."
- Terri Guillemets

"When it comes to eating right and exercising,
there is no 'I'll start tomorrow'.
Tomorrow is disease."
- Terri Guillemets

"When health is absent, wisdom cannot reveal itself,
art cannot manifest, strength cannot fight,
wealth becomes useless,
and intelligence cannot be applied."
- Herophilus

"Life can pull you down,
but running always lifts you up."
- Jenny Hadfield

"Living in the Moment could be the meaning of life."
- Jenny Hadfield

"Music is therapy. Music moves people.
It connects people in ways that no other medium can.
It pulls heart strings. It acts as medicine."
- Ben William Haggerty (aka Macklemore)

"America's health care system is in crisis precisely because
we systematically neglect wellness and prevention."
- Tom Harkin

"If we are serious about combating the childhood
obesity epidemic and improving child nutrition,
then everyone must chip in -
parents, schools, and yes even Congress."
- Tom Harkin

"Let's face it, in America today
we don't have a health care system,
we have a sick care system."
- Tom Harkin

"Parents should know that our schools are now
one of the largest sources of unhealthy food for their kids."
- Tom Harkin

"This study shows that when it comes to diet and obesity,
American parents are woefully uninformed."
- Tom Harkin

"Would anyone advocate that we take the fences
off the playground for elementary schools
and just let kids run around in the streets?...
By the same token, why would we allow schools
to sort of poison our kids with junk food?"
- Tom Harkin

"For me, working out is a form of therapy.
It's cathartic for me; it's a good stress reliever.
I know that when I go to the gym I am taking care of myself,
and I know I'll feel so much better afterwards."
- Bob Harper

"I believe in the power of the human spirit."
- Bob Harper

"I found that people like rules,
and I love to tell people what to do.
It's not rocket science when it comes to weight loss.
It's about eating a little less
and moving a little bit more."
- Bob Harper

"Whether you want to lose 20 pounds or 200,
what the contestants on 'The Biggest Loser'
have learned - and taught me holds true:
You've got to make a break.
You've got to divorce yourself from the past
and find a different way of living.
And you can never go back."
- Bob Harper

"You can't be a parent and say,
'I need you to be more active and I need you to eat right,'
when you're still choosing to have poor eating habits."
- Bob Harper

"Being in control of your life
and having realistic expectations
about your day-to-day challenges are
the keys to stress management,
which is perhaps the most important ingredient
to living a happy, healthy and rewarding life."
- Marilu Henner

"Foods high in bad fats, sugar and chemicals are
directly linked to many negative emotions,
whereas whole, natural foods rich in nutrients -
foods such as fruits, vegetables, grains and legumes -
contribute to greater energy and positive emotions."
- Marilu Henner

"I eat all of the time... at least five little meals a day."
- Marilu Henner

"I like getting up early. I get up around five."
- Marilu Henner

"It is now common knowledge
that the average American gains 7 pounds
between Thanksgiving and New Year's Day."
- Marilu Henner

"Often when a person can't get past stress,
she will turn to overeating, drinking or smoking,
which can become a greater problem than the stress itself."
- Marilu Henner

"Research has shown that even small amounts
of processed food alter the chemical balance
in our brain and cause negative mood swings
along with noticeable dips ill energy."
- Marilu Henner

"The biggest reason most people fail is that
they try to fix too much at once -
join a gym, get out of debt,
floss after meals and have thinner thighs in 30 days."
- Marilu Henner

"A wise man should consider that health is the greatest
of human blessings,
and learn how by his own thought
to derive benefit from his illnesses."
- Hippocrates

"If we could give every individual the right amount
of nourishment and exercise,
not too little and not too much,
we would have found the safest way to health."
- Hippocrates

"Natural forces within us are the true healers of disease."
- Hippocrates

"Walking is man's best medicine."
- Hippocrates

"Whenever a doctor cannot do good,
he must be kept from doing harm."
- Hippocrates

"Find a workout you love that you want to be better at.
Instead of focusing on how many pounds you're losing,
you can focus on improving your performance,
and you'll find happiness through that journey."
- Cassey Ho

"I realize now that I am not just an instructor at a gym,
but that I am a role model and leader in the fitness industry.
It is my responsibility to do whatever I can
to help people get healthier while
feeling confident and happy in their body."
- Cassey Ho

"It's not all about the scale.
It's about what you're made of!"
- Cassey Ho

"Not everyone has to be a runner or a crossfitter.
If dancing is your thing, join a dance class
and you'll find that you're getting a
great workout without feeling like it's a chore."
- Cassey Ho

"When you feel good, you feel that you look good,
and then you perform even better.
It's an amazing cycle."
- Cassey Ho

"At the surface, many people's goals are
to lose weight, tone up, feel better, etc.
But superficial goals get superficial results that usually fade.
Dig a little deeper, and the 'why' is usually unveiled:
to be more confident, to be more happy, to feel sexy again."
- Brett Hoebel

"Don't strive for perfection. It doesn't exist.
Strive for a better you. That's always in reach."
- Brett Hoebel

"Food is a lot of people's therapy -
when we say comfort food, we really mean that.
It's releasing dopamine and serotonin
in your brain that makes you feel good."
- Brett Hoebel

"If you think of exercise as a 60-minute commitment
3 times a week at the gym,
you're missing the point completely.
If you think that going on a diet
has something to do with nutrition,
you don't see the forest through the trees.
It is a lifestyle. I know it sounds cliche,
but you have to find things you love to do."
- Brett Hoebel

"If I could give one tip for people -
it's not an exercise or nutrition regimen.
It's to walk your talk and believe in yourself,
because at the end of the day,
the dumbbell and diet don't get you in shape.
It's your accountability to your word."
- Brett Hoebel

"If you don't have an emotional connection
to why you are trying to accomplish your goals,
the odds are you won't reach them or will quit trying."
- Brett Hoebel

"My approach to training changed dramatically throughout
my experience as one of the trainers on 'The Biggest Loser'.
Getting to know each person was an important reminder
that to get the body physically fit,
you must first get mentally and emotionally fit."
- Brett Hoebel

"Salt is one of the flavors that makes food taste good
- salt, sugar and fat.
So it's a natural thing for all chefs and cooks to add salt,
because it enhances the flavor of the food.
If you go out to eat, I guarantee
you're going to be eating a lot of salted foods
that you are going to have no idea."
- Brett Hoebel

"When it comes to sticking to your resolutions,
research has shown that 'action-oriented' resolutions
have a better chance of being upheld than 'idea-oriented'.
For example, a resolution to lose weight is really only an idea
with nothing actionable to do.
However, sticking with that goal in mind,
you could make the resolution action-oriented by saying
'get up 30 minutes earlier every Monday,
Wednesday and Friday and do a 20-minute
workout at home before work'.
Now you have an actionable path
on how to achieve your goal."
- Brett Hoebel

"You need to put what you learn into practice
and do it over and over again until it's a habit.
I always say, 'Seeing is not believing. Doing is believing.'
There is a lot to learn about fitness, nutrition and emotions,
but once you do, you can master them
instead of them mastering you."
- Brett Hoebel

"In our fast-forward culture,
we have lost the art of eating well.
Food is often little more than fuel to pour down the hatch
while doing other stuff - surfing the Web,
driving, walking along the street.
Dining al desko is now the norm in many workplaces.
All of this speed takes a toll.
Obesity, eating disorders and poor nutrition are rife."
- Carl Honore

"Don't just kind of do it!"
- Tony Horton

"Do your best and forget the rest."
- Tony Horton

"If you have health, you probably will be happy,
and if you have health and happiness,
you have the wealth you need,
even if it is not all you want."
- Elbert Hubbard

"The health care system is really designed to
reward you for being unhealthy.
If you are a healthy person and work hard to be healthy,
there are no benefits."
- Mike Huckabee

"We don't have a health care crisis,
we have a health crisis!"
- Mike Huckabee

"The groundwork of all happiness is health."
- Leigh Hunt

"Children with obesity and diabetes live harder poorer lives,
they often don't finish school and earn much less
than their healthy counterparts."
- Mark Hyman

"I don't need the fillers, additives, excessive amounts of sugars,
fats, salts and other measures taken to taint
the natural goodness of real food."
- Mark Hyman

"It seems that for many the cure to acne
is at the end of their fork,
not in a prescription pad."
- Mark Hyman

"Lifestyle change and changes in diet work faster,
better and more cheaply than any medication
and are as effective or more effective than gastric bypass
without any side effects or long-term complications."
- Mark Hyman

"Most schools have only a microwave or deep fryer,
hardly the tools needed to feed our children real, fresh food."
- Mark Hyman

"My advice is to give up stevia, aspartame, sucralose,
sugar alcohols like xylitol and malitol,
and all of the other heavily-used
and marketed sweeteners unless you want
to slow down your metabolism,
gain weight, and become an addict."
- Mark Hyman

"Paradoxically Americans are becoming both more obese
and more nutrient deficient at the same time.
Obese children eating processed foods are nutrient depleted
and increasingly get scurvy and rickets,
diseases we thought were left behind
in the 19th and 20th centuries."
- Mark Hyman

"Part of my training was learning how to refer patients to
cardiologists for heart problems, gastroenterologists
for stomach issues, and rheumatologists for joint pain.
Given that most physicians were trained this way,
it's no wonder that the average Medicare patient has
six doctors and is on five different medications."
- Mark Hyman

"Placing too much emphasis on a yes/no diagnosis,
meaning you either have a disease or you don't,
can lead even the most well-meaning physicians to miss
underlying causes and early warning signs of illness."
- Mark Hyman

"Seems you can't outsmart Mother Nature."
- Mark Hyman

"Stay away from milk. It is nature's perfect food
- but only if you are a calf."
- Mark Hyman

"The best advice is to avoid foods
with health claims on the label,
or better yet avoid foods with labels in the first place."
- Mark Hyman

"The body maintains balance in only a handful of ways.
At the end of the day, disease occurs when
these basic systems are out of whack."
- Mark Hyman

"The food industry profits from providing poor quality foods
with poor nutritional value that people eat a lot of."
- Mark Hyman

"The very fact that we are having a national conversation
about what we should eat, that we are struggling
with the question about what the best diet is,
is symptomatic of how far we have strayed
from the natural conditions that gave rise to our species,
from the simple act of eating real, whole, fresh food."
- Mark Hyman

"The way most doctors practice
medicine right now isn't working."
- Mark Hyman

"When it becomes a revolutionary act to eat real food,
we are in trouble."
- Mark Hyman

"You can't exercise your way out of a bad diet."
- Mark Hyman

"The good-news stories in medicine are
early detection, early intervention."
- Thomas R. Insel

"Health is a state of complete harmony
of the body, mind and spirit.
When one is free from physical disabilities
and mental distractions, the gates of the soul open."
- B. K. Iyengar

"As much as we pump iron and we run to build our strength up,
we need to build our mental strength up... so we can focus...
so we can be in concert with one another."
- Phil Jackson

"Burning fat is simple and straightforward
if you eat the foods we were built to eat
and get off the couch every once in a while.
There is hope."
- Abel James

"Grains rapidly elevate your blood sugar and cause
your body to store fat, rather than burn it.
How do you fatten a cow? Feed it grains.
How do you fatten a human? Feed it grains."
- Abel James

"If you can't pronounce an ingredient (or five) on the label,
you probably shouldn't eat it."
- Abel James

"In the United States, Big Food doesn't even have to tell you
which foods contain this genetically altered corn on the label or
whether it was used to feed the animals you're eating.
No wonder Europe won't import our food.
Even China, the country known for feeding poultry
feces to its farmed fish, banned our meat
and much of our processed food.
We can do better."
- Abel James

"It's important to note the few staples of the Standard American Diet
- namely corn, wheat, and soy are not produced in such
massive quantities because they're healthy.
They're produced because they make money for rich people."
- Abel James

"Modern food manufacturers have overwhelmed grocery store
shelves with foods that are nutrient poor, rotten, spoiled, dead, old,
and contaminated with antibiotics, chemicals, and growth hormones.
Refining has also brought us spectacularly cheap, pervasive,
and fattening ingredients: namely white flour, white sugar,
high fructose corn syrup, and industrial seed oils."
- Abel James

"One hundred years from now, medical doctors,
scientists, nutritionists, and the general public
will be puzzled and astounded by how few of us were
able to grasp the obvious - high-carb, low-fat diets
simply do not work long-term."
- Abel James

"Sure, it takes work to make (or find) fresh,
wild, natural food these days.
But the benefits for the health of our bodies
and the land we inhabit are undeniable.
- Abel James

"Leave all the afternoon for exercise and recreation,
which are as necessary as reading.
I will rather say more necessary
because health is worth more than learning."
- Thomas Jefferson

"Walking is the best possible exercise.
Habituate yourself to walk very far."
- Thomas Jefferson

"We never repent of having eaten too little."
- Thomas Jefferson

"Choose quality fuel: All calories are not equal.
1,500 calories of processed food has a completely
different effect on your body than 1,500 calories of fresh
fruits and vegetables, lean cuts of meat and whole grains.
The fiber and most of the nutrients are removed from most
processed foods like snack bars, crackers, bagels, chips,
bread, muffins and cereal, so when you eat these foods
your body recognizes them as sugar, spiking your insulin
and causing you to crave more food."
- Jeanette Jenkins

"Eat until you're satisfied and stop before you're full.
The stomach is made of smooth muscle,
and when you overeat you stretch the smooth muscle
of your stomach, which in turn increases your appetite.
Always stop eating as soon as you feel satisfied
to avoid stretching your stomach.
You can always eat again in two hours."
- Jeanette Jenkins

"Every living cell in your body is made from the food you eat.
If you consistently eat junk food
then you'll have a junk body."
- Jeanette Jenkins

"When you choose to perceive a situation in life,
you then have to live in that perception,
so if you choose to look for the negative,
then you will live in a negative experience,
and if you choose to look for the positive,
then you will live in a positive experience.
The choice is yours, so choose wisely."
- Jeanette Jenkins

"You can work out five times a week,
but if you're not eating a proper caloric intake,
then you will never achieve your goal weight.
You must make sure that you are eating fewer calories
than you are burning to continue with weight loss.
It sounds simple, yet most people have no idea
how many calories a day they eat and
never pay attention to portion control."
- Jeanette Jenkins

"You get out what you put in.
If you want more, give more."
- Jeanette Jenkins

"When a person goes into the operating room,
he will realize that there is one book
that he has yet to finish reading - 'Book of Healthy Life'."
- Steve Jobs

"All movement creates momentum.
All momentum is progress."
- Chalene Johnson

"If you consume just 100 calories more than you need a day,
you may very well gain as much as 10 pounds in a year."
- Chalene Johnson

"One common attribute of successful people is
they tend to exercise before they start their workday.
Successful people begin their day earlier than the rest.
They recognize that exercise enhances their
productivity and energy level."
- Chalene Johnson

"Positive energy is your priceless life force. Protect it.
Don't allow people to draw from your reserves;
select friends who recharge your energies...
I'm not asking you to cut people out of your life,
but I am asking you to invest your time with people
who will push you to be your best.
Winners love to see other people win."
- Chalene Johnson

"Resolve to do the things you find to be difficult.
That's what confident people do.
They tackle those things that are scary
and they get addicted to doing it."
- Chalene Johnson

"Successful people adopt the laws of success
by creating lifelong habits that become ingrained
and as much a part of who they are as the color of their
eyes. They don't have to think about it."
- Chalene Johnson

"The American College of Sports Medicine found that
the productivity of people after exercise was an average
of 65 percent higher than those who did not exercise.
If I have something that's really bothering me,
so much that it almost hurts my head to try to sort it out,
I always find the solution in a puddle of sweat!
Intense exercise is like taking a magic pill that
gives you the ability to solve problems like a superhero."
- Chalene Johnson

"The right habits are the only things that
separate you from the life you want to live."
- Chalene Johnson

"The vital difference between dreamers and achievers
boils down to some very basic, simple habits.
People with clear, 'written-out' goals who consistently honor
Their defined priorities tend to get results faster than others,
and enjoy a greater level of happiness and long-term
success in all areas of life.
Yet most of us have never been formally taught
a system of goal-setting and mastery that
can be applied to health and fitness."
- Chalene Johnson

"Treat yourself like a fat person with aches and pains
and a suitcase full of excuses, and good luck
- you'll stay exactly where you are.
Train like an athlete and, though you may
not look like one now, you will become one."
- Chalene Johnson

"When I hear health professionals suggesting that you
shouldn't worry about the balance of calories in
versus calories out, but rather eat clean and follow
your hunger instincts, well,
I really just want to pinch their heads off.
That's like a millionaire suggesting that instead of worrying
About what's in your bank account,
just listen to your shopping instincts
and buy high-quality goods …
weight loss is not magic.
To a great extent, it's accounting."
- Chalene Johnson

"Whether you believe you can lose the weight and
keep it off forever or that it probably won't happen for you,
either way, you're right!"
- Chalene Johnson

"Your health and fitness do not exist independently
of the other areas of your life."
- Chalene Johnson

"Your foundation determines your success."
- Chalene Johnson

"I make sure I get a lot of vegetables, a lot of fruit.
I am a big fruit man; I am a vegetable man, anyway."
- Earvin "Magic" Johnson Jr.

"The human body has been designed to resist
an infinite number of changes and attacks
brought about by its environment.
The secret of good health lies in successful adjustment
to changing stresses on the body."
- Harry J. Johnson

"Your body hears everything your mind says."
- Naomi Judd

"Make a list of what is really important to you. Embody it."
- Jon Kabat-Zinn

"Meditation is the only intentional,
systematic human activity
which at bottom is about not trying to improve yourself
or get anywhere else,
but simply to realize where you already are."
- Jon Kabat-Zinn

"Symptoms of illness and distress,
plus your feelings about them,
can be viewed as messengers coming to tell you something
important about your body or about your mind.
In the old days, if a king didn't like the message he was given,
he would sometimes have the messenger killed.
This is tantamount to suppressing your symptoms
or your feelings because they are unwanted.
Killing the messenger and denying the message
or raging against it are not intelligent ways
of approaching healing."
- Jon Kabat-Zinn

"We take care of the future best
by taking care of the present now."
- Jon Kabat-Zinn

"I can't provide you with the motivation to want to make
changes in your life -
that has to come from within you.
YOU have to decide that exercising
and eating healthy will be a priority in your life."
- Steve Kamb

"What we have in the United States is not so much a
health-care system as a disease-care system."
- Edward Kennedy

"Physical fitness is not only one of the most
important keys to a healthy body,
it is the basis of dynamic and
creative intellectual activity."
- John F. Kennedy

"I try my best to eat healthy the majority of the time
so that I feel good and have more energy.
I am so passionate about eating healthily,
I am actually certified in nutrition.
I try my best to eat organic whenever possible,
but it's important not to be too strict about it.
Just do the best you can."
- Miranda Kerr

"I've always had a burning desire to help people
and make a difference in the world.
I didn't know how I could do that in modeling
when it can be such a fake world.
But my dad told me I could make a difference
by being true to myself and teaching people
what I've learnt about spirituality, health and nutrition."
- Miranda Kerr

"There have been some good studies done in California with
Hispanic parents where in the course of a year,
they have changed their entire nutritional intake for the better.
The kid becomes, in a sense, the bridge
between the educational process and the home."
- C. Everett Koop

"When a child shows up for school,
and is not physically and mentally ready to learn,
he or she never catches up."
- C. Everett Koop

"Drinking freshly made juices and eating enough
whole foods to provide adequate fiber is a
sensible approach to a healthful diet."
- Jay Kordich

"Juicing is the key to a long, healthy,
disease-free life."
- Jay Kordich

"If everyone on a standard American diet
stopped eating cereal grains,
industrial seed oils, and excess sugar tomorrow,
I'm willing to bet that the rates of obesity, diabetes, heart disease,
and just about every chronic inflammatory disease
would plummet over the next decade."
- Chris Kresser

"Over the last several years I've come to believe that
chronic stress and the cascade of changes it causes in the body
is second only to diet as the primary cause of modern disease."
- Chris Kresser

"There is strong evidence to support the influence of
our food choices on the health and vibrancy of our skin."
- Chris Kresser

"A balanced life is like a three legged stool.
Each leg - nutrition, fitness and wellness
is necessary and supports the other."
- Ellie Krieger

"In my food world, there is no fear or guilt,
only joy and balance.
So no ingredient is ever off-limits.
Rather, all of the recipes here follow my
Usually-Sometimes-Rarely philosophy.
Notice there is no Never."
- Ellie Krieger

"I run 30 minutes in the morning,
and I'm literally the slowest person out there.
For example, just today, old people were speed-walking past me,
and I was like, 'This is pathetic,' but then I thought,
'I'm out here, I'm moving my body and I get to be outside'."
- Ellie Krieger

"I think that learning about nutrition transformed
my relationship with food in a healthy way."
- Ellie Krieger

"It's important to be aware of what we are eating,
but when we start to eat by numbers,
we lose something incredibly valuable,
which is enjoyment and pleasure."
- Ellie Krieger

"One of the biggest obstacles to reinventing your eating habits
is setting unrealistic goals.
Instead of saying, 'I'm never going to eat bread again',
take an objective step back,
and with loving intent, say to yourself,
'What can I realistically do and live with?'
If you are overly ambitious, it winds up backfiring,
which can be very painful
because you feel like you've failed."
- Ellie Krieger

"So often, people's perceptions of healthy food is that
there must be some compromise in taste and enjoyment,
but I try to show that it is all interconnected,
that delicious food can also be healthy food."
- Ellie Krieger

"There's no point in putting a value judgment on how good or bad you are based on how you're eating at any particular instant."
- Ellie Krieger

"To get people to eat well,
Don't say a word about health,
Just cook fantastic food for them."
- Ellie Krieger

"It is no measure of health to be well adjusted
to a profoundly sick society."
- J Krishnamurti

"There's more to life than training,
but training is what puts more in your life."
- Brooks Kubik

"When I cook with my son, I might chop vegetables
and have fun with different shapes.
Cooking is a way to teach kids about other things,
like reading or math with all of the weights and measures.
There are so many things that are part of cooking
that are also very educational."
- Emeril Lagasse

"I do it as a therapy. I do it as something to keep me alive.
We all need a little discipline.
Exercise is my discipline."
- Jack LaLanne

"Look at the average American diet:
ice cream, butter, cheese, whole milk, all this fat.
People don't realize how much of this stuff you
get by the end of the day.
High blood pressure is from all this high-fat eating."
- Jack LaLanne

"Probably millions of Americans got up this morning
with a cup of coffee, a cigarette and a donut.
No wonder they are sick and fouled up."
- Jack LaLanne

"The only way you get that fat off
is to eat less and exercise more."
- Jack LaLanne

"Yes, exercise is the catalyst.
That's what makes everything happen:
your digestion, your elimination, your sex life, your skin, hair,
everything about you depends on circulation.
And how do you increase circulation?"
- Jack LaLanne

"You don't have to call it God or Jesus.
That's religious humbug to a lot of people,
but you've gotta believe that nature
and spiritual things surround us.
That is what put us here!
I thank the universe for that every day of my life."
- Jack LaLanne

"No one has ever drowned in his own sweat."
- Ann Landers

"I run six-to-eight miles a day,
plus weights and aerobics in the lunch hour."
- Hugh Laurie

"Frequent self-weighing is one successful component
of maintaining long-term weight loss."
- Sohee Lee

"Ladies in particular:
I urge you to set performance goals in the gym.
Shoot for one strict bodyweight pull up.
Train for a powerlifting meet!
Learn a new skill, such as how to double clean kettlebells.
Doing so will allow you to feel truly empowered,
and you'll learn that true fitness success comes when
you fall in love with the process and enjoy the ride."
- Sohee Lee

"Many folks who like to demonize flexible dieting
overlook the fact that quality of life matters and that
a freakin' donut every now and then is perfectly okay."
- Sohee Lee

"When we are properly educated, the scale weight can actually be
an incredibly valuable tool to gauge health and fitness progress.
Frequent self-monitoring can improve self-awareness by alerting
the individual to subtle weight increases that can then
be nipped in the bud via dietary and exercise intervention."
- Sohee Lee

"Scientists have proven that it's impossible to long-jump 30 feet,
but I don't listen to that kind of talk.
Thoughts like that have a way of sinking into your feet."
- Carl Lewis

"Track and field is the best way to reach out for kids.
It doesn't matter how fast you are.
You always want to beat someone."
- Carl Lewis

"And in the end, it's not the years in your life that count.
It's the life in your years."
- Abraham Lincoln

"Don't be frustrated by comparing yourself
and your results to 20 yr. olds at the gym.
Being older you will become frustrated.
Instead compare yourself to those your age.
I promise you that your confidence and results will increase."
- Tom Link

"Don't let people who don't get the fitness lifestyle
sway you in any way.
It's OK to forgo happy hour to get your workout in."
- Tom Link

"I workout for what it does to my mind.
My physique is just a bi-product of
all of my hard work in the gym."
- Tom Link

"Make your default mode one of generosity.
It's a nice way to live, and it's contagious."
- Frank Lipman

"When you switch the lens and heal your mind of negativity,
it actually helps heal your body of exhaustion, aches, and pains."
- Frank Lipman

"To insure good health:
eat lightly, breathe deeply, live moderately,
cultivate cheerfulness, and maintain an interest in life."
- William Londen

"We are the authors of our own lives;
it falls only to us."
- Rob Lowe

"I'm a vegetarian, and I long for people to eat less meat,
but the thing to do is not to go, 'Eat! Less! Meat!' It's to say,
'I am fit as a flea and I'm 63, I haven't eaten meat for 40 years,
and I never get diseases, I'm never ill, and I'm full of energy.
So how's about that?"
- Joanna Lumley

"The greatest miracle on Earth is the human body.
It is stronger and wiser than you may realize,
and improving its ability to self heal is within your control."
- Fabrizio Mancini

"I promise you nothing is as chaotic as it seems.
Nothing is worth your health.
Nothing is worth poisoning yourself
into stress, anxiety, and fear."
- Steve Marabodi

"The greatest wealth is health."
- Publius Vergilius Maro (aka Virgil)

"Life is not merely being alive, but being well."
- Marcus Valerius Martialis

"I'd love to open up sessions at a Boys and Girls Club
or something where kids can learn nutrition
and how to exercise in a fun way.
Especially for young guys. I'd love to be an inspiration."
- James Maslow

"The aim of medicine is to prevent disease and prolong life,
the ideal of medicine is to eliminate the need of a physician."
- William J. Mayo

"Cook what's fresh for the day.
When you're using fresh fruits, vegetables, and foods,
it's easier to keep the weight off.
And I eat whatever I want - just not a ton of it."
- Debi Mazar

"All the money in the world can't buy you back good health."
- Reba McEntire

"Where your mind goes....your life goes.
Chart the course for your future by the thoughts
you think about in your mind.
Get in agreement with God and think positive
because when you do,
amazing things will happen in your life
and the lives of those around you!"
- Laura Thompson McFaden

"If we went back to the basics of vegetables, legumes, grains
- the things closer to the earth,
it's a lot better for the earth and for other people.
We can feed more people,
we can feed the starving people."
- Nellie McKay

"I've never dieted in my life; I like food too much.
I'm just thoughtful about what I eat,
and I'm lucky that I love the taste of vegetables.
I'm certainly not 'actress skinny,' and I never will be.
I'm strong, and my body works great for me."
- Sarah McLachlan

"Everyday I plant seeds in the Garden of My Dreams!
Cultivating passion and drive to live my Best Self:
Mind, 'Body', & Spirit."
- Ginny Scales Medeiros

"Health and intellect are the two blessings of life."
- Menander

"Eating foods that are in season will not only allow you
to enjoy tastier, fresher, and more available foods,
they may contain more nutrients, too."
- Joseph Mercola

"Food addiction is VERY real."
- Joseph Mercola

"Having a positive outlook and a cheerful disposition
isn't only a happier way to live your life
- it's a healthier way as well."
- Joseph Mercola

"I'm an advocate for the truth, and the truth is that,
every year, we are spending over $2 trillion in the U.S. alone
for a fatally-flawed health care system that is killing
hundreds of thousands of people every year,
simply because they do not have the understanding,
an awareness, of the alternatives to
potentially-toxic and expensive medications."
- Joseph Mercola

"Mindfulness and meditation are among the
best methods to boost your ability to focus.
Ideally, start your day with a mindfulness 'exercise,'
such as focusing on your breathing for five minutes
before you get out of bed.
This can help you to stay better focused
for the rest of your day."
- Joseph Mercola

"One of the best ways to prevent global disaster,
save our health, and build a sustainable economy is through
regenerative, sustainable agriculture."
- Joseph Mercola

"The connection between optimism and other positive emotions
and good health has been firmly established by scientific research,
and the link appears to be particularly strong when it comes to
heart health. Being lighthearted, it turns out,
is one of the best ways to protect your heart."
- Joseph Mercola

"If Americans alone reduced their meat consumption by just 10%,
it would free up enough land to grow 12 million tons of grain -
enough to save the six million children under the age of 5
that die every year as a result of hunger."
- Leilani Münter

"If I had to, you know, promote sugar water
or a candy bar in order to race a car,
I wouldn't race a car. So whenever I hit the race track,
my cars are carrying messages about issues that
I think are important, like renewable energies,
solar power, wind power."
- Leilani Münter

"I love doing hot yoga and it prepares me for the stamina
I need to be in a race car for long periods of time."
- Leilani Münter

"Never underestimate a vegan hippie chick with a race car."
- Leilani Münter

"I believe that the greatest gift you can give
your family and the world is a healthy you."
- Joyce Meyer

"It's so important to realize that every time you get upset,
it drains your emotional energy. Losing your cool makes you tired.
Getting angry a lot messes with your health."
- Joyce Meyer

"There's no happier person than a truly thankful, content person."
- Joyce Meyer

"You cannot have a positive life and a negative mind."
- Joyce Meyer

"It's so important to realize that every time you get upset,
it drains your emotional energy. Losing your cool makes you tired.
Getting angry a lot messes with your health."
- Joyce Meyer

"I've always believed fitness is an entry point to
help you build that happier, healthier life.
When your health is strong, you're capable of taking risks.
You'll feel more confident to ask for the promotion.
You'll have more energy to be a better mom.
You'll feel more deserving of love."
- Jillian Michaels

"My agenda is trying to help people live a better life."
- Jillian Michaels

"Respect your body. Eat well. Dance forever."
- Eliza Gaynor Minden

"The torch relay is an excellent embodiment of all that
the Olympic Gameshave come to symbolize
- a celebration of the human spirit.
Personally to me, it represents striving to be the best
in whatever we do, never giving up despite the odds,
and a commitment to health and fitness."
- Lakshmi Mittal

"Some coaches are not educated at the elite level
in health and nutrition.
They're not educated in how the body works
from anatomy and physiology perspectives."
- Dominique Moceanu

"The mind has great influence over the body,
and maladies often have their origin there."
- Jean Baptiste Molière

"I love the idea of getting up early on Sundays and
walking to the market to pick up fresh fruits and vegetables.
It's a good way to start my day, and it makes me feel like
I've accomplished something before other people are even awake."
- Mandy Moore

"Every night I watch the nightly news.
It's funded by the pharmaceutical companies.
Virtually every ad is a drug ad. They get their say every night
on the nightly news through advertising."
- Michael Moore

"If you're in a diabetic or pre-diabetic state,
it's good to have medication to go on for a period of time.
But simply by making the changes - get your sleep,
35 grams of fiber and a half-hour walk -
your cholesterol will come down,
your sugar will come down,
and your blood pressure will come down.
Only the minority of people can't control it."
- Michael Moore

"The number 1 cause of bankruptcies is medical bills."
- Michael Moore

"Health messages are simply overwhelmed,
in volume and in effectiveness,
by junk-food ads that often deploy celebrities
or cartoon characters to great effect.
We may know that eating fruits and vegetables is good for us,
but the preponderance of the signals we get
- and especially the signals children get
push us in the direction of junk food."
- Michael Moss

"Because I'm a chef, I eat out frequently, so it's hard
for me to control what I consume in terms of calories.
But when I'm at home, I eat what my wife cooks for me.
She works hard to avoid making foods that are
high in calories and cholesterol, so most of the time,
she makes vegetarian dishes."
- Masaharu Morimoto

"I'm at the gym at 6, so I'm usually in my office by 7:15.
And I try to not schedule a lot of meetings before 8.
So I've got that first hour to get myself organized for the day
and to make sure that I've structured what I want to do."
- Anne M. Mulcahy

"Investing in early childhood nutrition is a surefire strategy.
The returns are incredibly high."
- Anne M. Mulcahy

"By eating many fruits and vegetables in place of
fast food and junk food, people could avoid obesity."
- David H. Murdock

"No pills, not even aspirin, and certainly no supplements
ever enter my mouth - everything I need comes from
my fish and vegetarian diet, which incorporates many
different kinds of fruit and vegetables every week."
- David H. Murdock

"Healthy, sustainable food production methods give us food
that is nutritionally better and with fewer pesticides,
antibiotics, and hormones."
- Marion Nestle

"I am not a vegetarian. I subscribe to my own mantra:
eat less, move more, eat plenty of fruits and vegetables,
don't eat too much junk food, and enjoy what you eat.
Or, to summarize: eat less, eat better,
move more, and get political."
- Marion Nestle

"I have a generally optimistic temperament and am thrilled
by what I see as a rapidly growing food movement,
especially among young people
who care about how food is produced
and what it does to their health and the environment."
- Marion Nestle

"It's time to get the FDA to reverse its 1994 decision
not to label GM foods."
- Marion Nestle

"Going meat-free can make a huge difference.
Studies show that vegetarians are, on average,
10 to 20 pounds lighter than meat-eaters and that
a vegetarian diet reduces our risk of heart disease
by 40 percent and adds seven or more years to our lifespan."
- Ingrid Newkirk

"Real nutrition comes from soybeans, almonds, rice,
and other healthy vegetable sources, not from a cow's udder."
- Ingrid Newkirk

"We are living in a world today where lemonade
is made from artificial flavors
and furniture polish is made from real lemons."
- Alfred Newman

"I live every day to its fullest extent and
I don't sweat the small stuff."
- Olivia Newton-John

"I'm happy, and I think being happy
keeps you looking young."
- Olivia Newton-John

"I've always been aware of my health
- when you are having to go on stage and perform,
you need to be feeling good
- but when I was diagnosed with a life-threatening illness,
I became really, really conscious of my health."
- Olivia Newton-John

"Growing Old Is Inevitable. Aging Is Optional!"
- Christiane Northrup

"If you are constantly around negativity,
that will adversely affect you."
- Christiane Northrup

"Joy is contagious and amplifies everything else that goes on."
- Christiane Northrup

"People with the most varied social contact have the best immunity."
- Christiane Northrup

"So much of what we are is about our programming.
What we think about, we focus on;
what we focus on can manifest."
- Christiane Northrup

"And let's be clear: It's not enough just to limit ads
for foods that aren't healthy.
It's also going to be critical to increase marketing
for foods that are healthy."
- Michelle Obama

"Choose people who lift you up."
- Michelle Obama

"Exercise is really important to me - it's therapeutic.
So if I'm ever feeling tense or stressed or like
I'm about to have a meltdown,
I'll put on my iPod and head to the gym or
out on a bike ride along Lake Michigan with the girls."
- Michelle Obama

"I look at how my kids view exercise.
They have a complete understanding
that nutrition and exercise go hand in hand.
I didn't think like that when I was a kid.
But they have a real consciousness about it
that I'd like to think comes from the years
of attention we've put into this."
- Michelle Obama

"The problem is when that fun stuff becomes the habit.
And I think that's what's happened in our culture.
Fast food has become the everyday meal."
- Michelle Obama

"We can make a commitment to promote vegetables and fruits
and whole grains on every part of every menu.
We can make portion sizes smaller and
emphasize quality over quantity.
And we can help create a culture - imagine this
where our kids ask for healthy options
instead of resisting them."
- Michelle Obama

"When I get up and work out, I'm working out
just as much for my girls as I am for me,
because I want them to see a mother who loves them dearly,
who invests in them, but who also invests in herself.
It's just as much about letting them know
as young women that it is okay to put yourself
a little higher on your priority list."
- Michelle Obama

"Every forkful of what you put in your mouth is either
inflammatory or anti-inflammatory. Make wise choices."
- Tom O'Bryan

"The World Health Organization tells us the United States ranks
second in overall health care... second from the bottom."
- Tom O'Bryan

"An unhealthy life is no life at all!"
- Kim Oexner

"Health is a unity of mind, body and soul!"
- Kim Oexner

"Without Health there is no Wealth!"
- Kim Oexner

"A rewarding life is based on your health!"
- Larry Oexner

"Health is wealth."
- Larry Oexner

"No pill manufactured can replace the warmth
of the sun and the bounty of nature!"
- Larry Oexner

"Oexnercise with Dr. Oexner."
- Larry Oexner

"Our candle of life lasts just so long.
It is a flicker for some,
a bright shining beacon for others.
The foods we eat,
the physical activity we bestow upon ourselves
and the spiritual message we live by,
makes that candle a bit shorter or a bit longer!"
- Larry Oexner

"Your body is your temple.
Your Food is your martyr!"
- Larry Oexner

"I challenge you, to go to any school
and open 50 lunch boxes, and I guarantee you
there will be one or two cans of Red Bull,
there'll be cold McDonald's and jam sandwiches
with several cakes."
- Jamie Oliver

"Many kids can tell you about drugs but
do not know what celery or courgettes taste like."
- Jamie Oliver

"The public health of five million children
should not be left to luck or chance."
- Jamie Oliver

"Because the biological mechanisms that affect
our health and well-being are so dynamic,
when people change their diet and lifestyle,
they usually feel so much better, so quickly;
it reframes the reason for changing
from fear of dying to joy of living.
Also, the support that patients give
each other is a powerful motivator."
- Dean Ornish

"I grew up in Texas, eating meat five times a day,
and I liked meat. But I began being a vegetarian
when I was 19 because I found that I felt better."
- Dean Ornish

"People who are lonely and depressed are
three to 10 times more likely to get sick and die
prematurely than those who have
a strong sense of love and community.
I don't know any other single factor that affects our health
- for better and for worse - to such a strong degree."
- Dean Ornish

"Poor health is not caused by something you don't have;
it's caused by disturbing something that you already have.
Healthy is not something that you need to get,
it's something you have already if you don't disturb it."
- Dean Ornish

"Think about it: Heart disease and diabetes,
which account for more deaths in the U.S. and worldwide
than everything else combined, are completely preventable
by making comprehensive lifestyle changes.
Without drugs or surgery."
- Dean Ornish

"It is much more important to know what sort of a patient
has a disease than what sort of a disease a patient has."
- William Osler

"One of the first duties of the physician is to
educate the masses not to take medicine."
- William Osler

"The good physician treats the disease;
the great physician treats the patient who has the disease."
- William Osler

"A lot of psychological principles and even medical principles,
you see them coming around to what the Bible
said hundreds of years ago:
a merry heart is good like a medicine."
- Joel Osteen

"A lot of folks believe their best years are behind them.
But I want Americans to recognize that's not true."
- Mehmet Oz

"Every hour you sit at work increases your mortality 11 percent.
Think about that."
- Mehmet Oz

"Food is no longer sacred to us:
in becoming too efficient we've changed its nature."
- Mehmet Oz

"If I make your workplace conducive to walking at lunch,
or working out at some time during the day,
or I get people to use the stairs more by
creating incentives to do such,
then people will start doing it naturally."
- Mehmet Oz

"If you don't know your blood pressure,
it's like not knowing the value of your company."
- Mehmet Oz

"I get up at the same time every morning."
- Mehmet Oz

"I saw many people who had advanced heart disease
and I was so frustrated because I knew if they just knew
how to do the right thing,
simple lifestyle and diet steps,
that the entire trajectory of their life
and health would have been different."
- Mehmet Oz

"Most allopathic doctors think practitioners
of alternative medicine are all quacks.
They're not. Often they're sharp people
who think differently about disease."
- Mehmet Oz

"People say their weight is genetic.
But it turns out that people who are overweight
don't just have overweight kids.
They also have overweight pets. That's not genetic."
- Mehmet Oz

"The rule I use is, If it doesn't come out of the ground
looking the way it looks when you eat it, be careful."
- Mehmet Oz

"We are spending most of our time in American health care fixing
the mistakes that either we in the profession are causing or our
patients are, without recognizing it, causing to themselves."
- Mehmet Oz

"We don't need sugar to live,
and we don't need it as a society."
- Mehmet Oz

"We don't walk.
We overeat because we've made it easy to overeat.
We have fast-food joints on every corner.
By the way, the 'we' is all of us.
It's not the government. It's all of us doing this together."
- Mehmet Oz

"Your genetics load the gun.
Your lifestyle pulls the trigger."
- Mehmet Oz

"Ignore the scale,
and make the process your goal."
- Harley Pasternak

"You're eating right and exercising regularly.
But there is one barrier in the way to slimming down:
It's our sneaky old nemesis, sugar,
which lies in wait at every turn."
- Harley Pasternak

"If the whole world went vegan, there would be less war.
How you eat determines your mood and your outlook on life."
- Alexandra Paul

"Sometimes I wake up in the morning & go Ahh...
I don't want to work out!
But I do anyway, because I'll always feel better afterwards.
I have never once worked out & felt worse."
- Alexandra Paul

"I had the privilege of practicing medicine in the early '60s,
before we had any government.
It worked rather well, and there was nobody
on the street suffering with no medical care."
- Ron Paul

"You pray for good health and a
body that will be strong in old age.
Good - but your rich foods block the gods' answer
and tie Jupiter's hands."
- Persius

"Don't show up late.
Don't try to slide out early.
Don't cheat your rep counts.
And definitely, don't hold back.
Leave it all in the gym!"
- Gunnar Peterson

"I always advise eating regular meals -
a mix of healthy carbs, protein and fruits and veggies."
- Gunnar Peterson

"I am a big believer in taking responsibility for your actions.
I tell my kids every day to 'own it' –
'it' being whatever they've said or done.
At some point in your life, you are in charge.
You call the shots. You decide to eat or not eat.
Is lack of will power a disease? Is lack of self-discipline a disease?
I would love to eat my body weight in chocolate chip cookies,
french fries, and peanut butter, but I don't. I choose not to.
That's on me, just like it's on me if I choose to do it."
- Gunnar Peterson

"I think the AMA got this one wrong (labeling Obesity a 'disease')
and I think the repercussions are going to be ugly.
America wasn't made on blame; it was made on responsibility.
Take off the training wheels in life
and decide to take responsibility for your actions."
- Gunnar Peterson

"The first thing people lose on a diet is their sense of humor.
Keep it fun. Keep it light."
- Gunnar Peterson

"Youth has no age."
- Pablo Picasso

"Happiness is the true goal behind the things we do.
Don't ever let people hijack this goal from you."
- Brad Pilon

"I think if people's lives were a little more exciting they
wouldn't need to eat so much to get some joy out of their day."
- Brad Pilon

"I think the very point is to not let things like TV distract us.
So Eat when Hungry, not Eat when Bored.
Go to sleep when tired,
not Go to sleep when American Idol is over."
- Brad Pilon

"Attention to health is life's greatest hindrance."
- Plato

"Lack of activity destroys the good condition of every human being,
while movement and methodical physical exercise
save it and preserve it."
- Plato

"Every major food company now has an organic division.
There's more capital going into organic agriculture
than ever before."
- Michael Pollan

"Very simply, we subsidize high-fructose corn syrup
in this country, but not carrots.
While the surgeon general is raising alarms
over the epidemic of obesity,
the president is signing farm bills designed to
keep the river of cheap corn flowing,
guaranteeing that the cheapest calories
in the supermarket will continue to be the unhealthiest."
- Michael Pollan

"It's been said that people become like their friends,
loved ones, and associates (and even their pets!).
If you want to be healthy, you should hang out with
healthy people and absorb their energy.
If you want to be happy,
you should surround yourself with happy people."
- Chris Powell

"Small changes over time lead to
extraordinary long-term results!"
- Chris Powell

"The chief condition on which, life, health
and vigor depend on, is action.
It is by action that an organism develops its faculties,
increases its energy, and attains the fulfillment of its destiny."
- Colin Powell

"Get Moving Tip: Before going to bed, leave your running shoes
on your bathroom counter (or throw them in your gym bag!)
so they're the first thing you see in the morning.
Sometimes, that extra reminder to
get moving is the best motivator!"
- Heidi Powell

"As long as my body is in shape,
my mind is working at its full capacity."
- Victoria Principal

"I believe that how you feel is very important to how you look
- that healthy equals beautiful."
- Victoria Principal

"It is so easy to forget that this is good that we're alive.
We should be enjoying this gift of being alive."
- Victoria Principal

"Dance like there's nobody watching
Love like you'll never get hurt
Sing like there's nobody listening
Live like it's heaven on earth
And speak from the heart to be heard."
- William W. Purkey

"I'm nutty for nutrition.
I've become one of those people who
can't stop talking about the connection
between food and health.
Now that I know how much changing what you eat
can transform your life,
I can't stop proselytizing."
- Robin Quivers

"Drink always before thirst,
and it will never overtake you."
- Francois Rabelais

"Without health, life is not life;
it is only a state of languor and suffering."
- Francois Rabelais

"Live boldly, laugh loudly.
Play as often as you can."
- Mary Anne Radmacher

"I started running 3 miles every morning after throat surgery
to remove a cyst last year.
The gym used to be my adversary.
But that has all changed.
Now, I look forward to it every morning."
- Rachael Ray

"I've never been a huge sweets eater,
and I've always loved a Mediterranean diet.
We eat a lot of dark leafy greens,
and a couple meals each week are meat-free.
We enjoy eating a balanced diet."
- Rachael Ray

"The magazine, the daytime show,
we've always tried to write affordable, accessible.
Those are key words for us, and I do mean us,
a huge staff of people at the magazine who love to cook affordable,
friendly food that helps families eat better for less."
- Rachael Ray

"Life's a river, you gotta go where it takes you."
- Shiva Rea

"You can't 'take' a breath, your breath is given to you."
- Shiva Rea

"The patient should be made to understand that
he or she must take charge of his own life.
Don't take your body to the doctor as if he were a repair shop."
- Quentin Regestein

"No one is immune from obesity - it affects
everyone from every race, gender and age.
For the first time in history,
there is a real possibility that children
will not outlive their parents as a result of
weight-related illnesses and other diseases.
There has to be a better way!"
- Tosca Reno

"Put simply, Clean Eating is avoiding all processed food,
relying on fresh fruits, vegetables and whole grains
rather than prepackaged or fast food."
- Tosca Reno

"Remember that a healthy body is built or destroyed
one decision at a time. It's up to you."
- Tosca Reno

"Some of the most challenging moves towards health
are made with the simplest of steps and that is why
I wrote The Start Here Diet."
- Tosca Reno

"There is simply no other exercise, and certainly no machine,
that produces the level of central nervous system activity,
improved balance and coordination, skeletal loading and
bone density enhancement, muscular stimulation and growth,
connective tissue stress and strength,
psychological demand and toughness,
and overall systemic conditioning
than the correctly performed full squat."
- Mark Rippetoe

"Alkalize and Energize!"
- Anthony Robbins

"Motion creates emotion."
- Anthony Robbins

"Now, more than ever, busy lifestyles, stress,
easy access to fast foods,
exposure to toxic chemicals,
and a diminished quality of our food supply
require that we take control and actively pursue the health,
energy and vitality we all desire and deserve now."
- Anthony Robbins

"Nothing tastes as good as excellent health."
- Anthony Robbins

"Remember: If you just keep doing
what you have always been doing,
you're going to have the energy you've always had.
No more, no less."
- Anthony Robbins

"The higher your energy level, the more efficient your body.
The more efficient your body, the better you feel
And the more you will use your talent
to produce outstanding results."
- Anthony Robbins

"The only people without problems are those in cemeteries."
- Anthony Robbins

"The quality of your life is dependent upon the
quality of the life of your cells.
If the bloodstream is filled with waste products,
the resulting environment does not promote a strong, vibrant,
healthy cell life-or biochemistry capable of
creating a balanced emotional life for an individual."
- Anthony Robbins

"Want to learn to eat a lot? Here it is: Eat a little.
That way, you will be around long enough to eat a lot."
- Anthony Robbins

"We all know that without our health,
nothing else matters."
- Anthony Robbins

"What good is having powerful goals
if you don't have the energy to carry them out?"
- Anthony Robbins

"Where focus goes, energy flows."
- Anthony Robbins

"Your daily decisions can either keep you
from achieving the body you desire -
or create the body you've always dreamed of."
- Anthony Robbins

"Awareness is bad for the meat business.
Conscience is bad for the meat business.
Sensitivity to life is bad for the meat business.
DENIAL, however, the meat business finds indispensable."
- John Robbins

"Few of us are aware that the act of eating
can be a powerful statement of commitment
to our own well-being, and at the same time the
creation of a healthier habitat.
Your health, happiness, and the future of life on earth
are rarely so much in your own hands
as when you sit down to eat."
- John Robbins

"I believe that eating simple food in a healthy body
with a clean conscience is more pleasurable,
and infinitely more satisfying, then eating decadent food
that makes you and your world ill."
- John Robbins

"Meat production is the second or third largest contributor to
environmental problems at every level and at every scale,
from global to local.
It is a primary culprit in land degradation,
air pollution, water shortage, water pollution,
species extinction, loss of biodiversity, and climate change."
- John Robbins

"The fork is the most powerful tool
ever placed in our hands."
- John Robbins

"The joy is that we can take back our bodies,
reclaim our health, and restore ourselves to balance.
We can take power over what and how we eat.
We can rejuvenate and recharge ourselves,
bringing healing to the wounds we carry inside us,
and bringing to fuller life
the wonderful person that each of us can be."
- John Robbins

"There is a reason why more than forty insurance companies
now cover all or part of the Ornish program.
Nearly 80 percent of patients with severely
clogged arteries who follow the Ornish program
for a year or more are able to avoid bypass or angioplasty.
Despite (or maybe because of) such outstanding results,
the Ornish program has been the subject of massive controversy.
Some say his approach is too drastic,
and we should stick to more medically conservative methods.
Ornish's reply is simple and difficult to argue with:
'I don't understand why asking people to eat
a well-balanced vegetarian diet is considered drastic,
while it's medically conservative to cut people open or put them
on powerful cholesterol-lowering drugs for the rest of their lives'."
- John Robbins

"You know that a majority of the medical costs
that are bankrupting families, companies,
and nations could be eliminated with better nutrition."
- John Robbins

"Buy direct from farmers. When you join a CSA
(Community Supported Agriculture),
you enter into a direct win-win partnership with local farmers."
- Ocean Robbins

"Cut down on animal products.
Approximately one-third of the calories consumed
by people living in developed nations are from animal sources.
Animal foods - like meat, poultry, fish, milk, and cheese
are usually an expensive source of protein and nutrients."
- Ocean Robbins

"Grow food. It takes time, but gardening is the
most economical way to enjoy the freshest possible food."
- Ocean Robbins

"Healthy food is a fundamental building block for a healthy life."
- Ocean Robbins

"Use what's in season, economical and nutritious.
Some of the most budget-conscious starches include
beans, whole grains, and potatoes.
Some of the most affordable and nutritionally potent vegetables
often include cabbage, carrots, and onions."
- Ocean Robbins

"Take care of your body.
It's the only place you have to live."
- Jim Rohn

"Four studies, all reported in the last five years,
have found what many suspected all along:
that a positive attitude makes a large difference
in how long and how well you live."
- Michael F. Roizen

"If any food has any one of the five ingredients below as any one
of the first five ingredients on the label, don't let it near your mouth.
1) Simple sugars
2) Enriched, bleached, or refined flour
(this means it's stripped of its nutrients)
3) All syrups, including HFCS
(high-fructose corn syrup—a four-letter word)
4) Saturated fat
(four-legged animal fat or palm or coconut oil)
5) Trans fat
(partially hydrogenated vegetable oil)."
- Michael F. Roizen

"In fact, behavioral choices account almost entirely for
a person's overall health and longevity by age sixty.
The older you are, the more your choices determine
how long and how well you live."
- Michael F. Roizen

"To help curb hunger and avoid binge eating,
drink a glass or two of water before you eat."
- Michael F. Roizen

"Walk thirty minutes a day and build a little muscle.
When you lose some weight,
your cells become more sensitive
and responsive to leptin."
- Michael F. Roizen

"A big barrier to getting people to eat
more fruits and vegetables
is convenience, the packaging and accessibility."
- Barbara Rolls

"I think it's quite obvious we need innovative strategies
to limit the impact of portion size on intake."
- Barbara Rolls

"People like value. We've got to shift people away
from this value way of thinking
of simply getting the most calories for the least dollars,
to value in terms of health."
- Barbara Rolls

"Be consistent: It's not about how much you do
in a given workout or how hard it is.
Ten minutes of core exercises four to five times per week
is far better than one long run a week."
- Rich Roll

"Don't diet: Instead, get honest about your habits and embark
on implementing healthy, lasting changes in your nutrition.
I feel quite strongly that a nutrition program built
entirely around plant-based foods and completely
devoid of animal products is optimal."
- Rich Roll

"It's crazy how emotional and threatened people
can become when the subject turns to food and diet.
Merely mentioning plant-based nutrition
often prompts immediate debate.
But I relish the dialogue. It's been a kick confronting
head-on the arguments of the critics
and dissenting voices and putting them to the test.
I've done my homework. I know how I feel.
And my results speak for themselves."
- Rich Roll

"Let's join together to shift the world's perspective
on long-term health and wellness.
No matter how old, overweight or out of shape you are,
you have the power to make a decision,
set a goal and create a plan.
Positive change is always within your grasp,
and today still remains the first day of the rest of your life.
Make it count!
- Rich Roll

"Let's wrap up the protein question
with one thought to ponder.
Some of the strongest and most fierce animals
in the world are Plant Powered.
The elephant, rhino, hippo, and gorilla
have one thing in common -
they all get 100 percent of their protein from plants."
- Rich Roll

"Nothing changes if nothing changes."
- Rich Roll

"Remember that its not about the result
- it's about the journey."
- Rich Roll

"The prize never goes to the fastest guy.
It goes to the guy who slows down the least.
True in endurance sports.
And possibly even truer in life."
- Rich Roll

"Ultra marathon legend and plant-strong Scott Jurek
claims that his body has become so adept at absorbing
his nutrient rich foods that he needs to eat less
and operates at a higher efficiency.
I can honestly say that I know what he is talking about.
And I think he and Carl Lewis
(who performed at his peak on a plant-based diet)
know what they are talking about."
- Rich Roll

"When it comes to exercise, it shouldn't be too painful.
Ideally, it should be fun. If you absolutely hate running,
find something else you enjoy. Otherwise, you set yourself up to fail.
And don't be too rigid - mix it up with a variety of activities
you like to keep it interesting and fresh."
- Rich Roll

"When the mind is controlled and spirit aligned with purpose,
the body is capable of so much more than we realize."
- Rich Roll

"Buy the jeans that make your ass look the nicest."
- John Romaniello

"Floss your teeth for better fitness."
- John Romaniello

"Get your clothes tailored.
A 200-dollar suit that fits well looks better
than a 500-dollar suit that doesn't."
- John Romaniello

"If getting a great body was easy,
every woman would look like Jessica Biel,
and every guy would have a body like Kellan Lutz."
- John Romaniello

"It's not the years in your life; it's the life in your years.
Don't listen to arguments on lifestyle based on longevity.
For me, living a life fully of *quality* years is by far more important
than making sure I have a higher total quantity of them.
I quantify that quality by feelings of enjoying my food,
loving the way I look, and achieving my goals."
- John Romaniello

"Learn how to cook.
If you're approaching 30 and you
can't make a few meals,
take the next month and learn."
- John Romaniello

"Never get more than 9 hours of sleep, or less than 3.
I believe in adequate rest,
but too much sleep wasting time
That could be spent on anything from
self-edification to world domination."
- John Romaniello

"The best training program in the world is
absolutely worthless without the will to
execute it properly, consistently, and with intensity."
- John Romaniello

"Use your sex drive as a general measure of health,
as it indicates hormonal balance.
Low sex drive is a symptom of everything from
depression to low testosterone to over-training."
- John Romaniello

"Believe in YOU so much that people
will jump on YOUR BANDWAGON."
- Martin Rooney

"Challenges will happen. What's the lesson?
The Black Belt isn't the guy that doesn't make any mistakes.
It's the guy that made all of them."
- Martin Rooney

"Of all the people on the planet,
you talk to yourself more than anyone.
Make sure you are saying the right things."
- Martin Rooney

"You will know if you are too acidic if you get sick often,
get urinary tract infections, suffer from headaches,
and have bad breath and body odor
(when you do not use antiperspirant).
Acidosis is the medical term for a blood alkalinity of less than 7.35.
A normal reading is called homeostasis.
It is not considered a disease;
although in and of itself it is
recognized as an indicator of disease."
- Natalia Rose

"Being lean is not normal in today's society.
This means you need to do things that normal people don't do.
You need to pack your own lunch; you need to request food be
prepared differently than what's listed on most menus;
your idea of 'fast food' should be a protein shake; and you
can't take the weekend off from your diet like you do your job."
- Mike Roussell

"High-fiber foods - such as vegetables,
fruits and whole grains - not only provide volume,
but also take longer to digest,
making you feel full longer."
- Mike Roussell

"Nowadays everyone is connected every second of everyday.
Cell phones, internet, email, TiVo, you know what I mean.
It is so important to unplug yourself.
Meditation is another great way to reduce stress and cortisol.
You don't have to become a monk or
anything but 20 minutes of sitting with no distractions
and focusing on your breathing will do wonders."
- Mike Roussell

"Nutrition doesn't have to be complicated;
in fact it is very simple.
Unfortunately nutrition is big business
so companies are always looking for
the next idea or concept they can tweak to make a buck."
- Mike Roussell

"70 percent of long-term gym memberships are mostly unused,
but a dog needs walking every day."
- Gretchen Rubin

"I should make one healthy choice, and then stop choosing."
- Gretchen Rubin

"Once the habit is in place,
we can effortlessly do the things we want to do."
- Gretchen Rubin

"The desire to start something at the 'right' time
is usually just a justification for delay.
In almost every case, the best time to start is now."
- Gretchen Rubin

"We all know the secret of dieting
- eat better, eat less, exercise more
- it's the application that's challenging."
- Gretchen Rubin

"What you do every day matters more
than what you do once in a while."
- Gretchen Rubin

"As places of learning, schools have a responsibility
to also educate on nutrition,
which we all can agree is far more important than algebra,
no matter what your third-period teacher claims."
- Lynda Resnick

"Motivation is what gets you started.
Habit is what keeps you going."
- Jim Ryun

"I was a vegetarian first.
I had high blood pressure at 27,
everybody in my family died of cancer,
and I knew it was in the food,
so I changed my diet."
- John Salley

"Children want to mimic adults.
They notice when you choose to prepare fresh vegetables
over calling in another pizza pie for dinner.
They will see that food made with love and care
Outweighs going through the drive-through window."
- Marcus Samuelsson

"Cooking with your kids and engaging them in hands-on activities
are two ways to begin to educate children about the healthy eating,
and kick start the important task to help change
how the younger generation looks at food and nutrition."
- Marcus Samuelsson

"Let the fresh fruits and vegetables be your guide,
and make something that will keep for the whole week."
- Marcus Samuelsson

"Nutrition doesn't have to be complicated.
It goes back to the lessons you learned as a kid.
Start with a real breakfast; don't ever skip that.
If you're waking up early for a run,
make sure you drink at least a glass of water
and put something healthy into your stomach
before you go out the door."
- Summer Sanders

"I'm simple. I love hiking, going to the gym,
doing some simple stuff. I love being outdoors,
I love bike riding. Just stuff that's fun!"
- Lea Michele Sarfati (aka Lea Michele)

"I was a vegan for two years, and I really enjoyed it.
Then, I got to a point in my life at which I wanted
to do something else, so now I'm a vegetarian.
You should make your diet one that best fits you
and how you feel. Listen to your body.
The most important thing is to exercise,
drink lots of water, and take really good care of yourself."
- Lea Michele Sarfati (aka Lea Michele)

"Looking after my health today gives me
a better hope for tomorrow."
- Anne Wilson Schaef

"We have finally started to notice that there is real curative value
in local herbs and remedies. In fact, we are also becoming aware
that there are little or no side effects to most natural remedies,
and that they are often more effective than Western medicine."
- Anne Wilson Schaef

"With sizeable muscles, you're carrying more weight,
which would be counterproductive to endurance performance,
it would be like running a long distance while carrying a suitcase."
- Brad Schoenfeld

"The greatest of follies is to sacrifice health
for any other kind of happiness."
- Arthur Schopenhauer

"I'm addicted to exercising and
I have to do something every day."
- Arnold Schwarzenegger

"It's simple, if it jiggles, it's fat."
- Arnold Schwarzenegger

"Strength does not come from winning.
Your struggles develop your strengths.
When you go through hardships
and decide not to surrender,
that is strength."
- Arnold Schwarzenegger

"The resistance that you fight physically in the gym
and the resistance that you fight in life
can only build a strong character."
- Arnold Schwarzenegger

"To be successful, you must dedicate yourself 100%
to your training, diet and mental approach."
- Arnold Schwarzenegger

"Training gives us an outlet for suppressed energies
created by stress and thus tones the spirit
just as exercise conditions the body."
- Arnold Schwarzenegger

"What we face may look insurmountable.
But I learned something from all those years
of training and competing.
I learned something from all those sets and reps
when I didn't think I could lift another ounce of weight.
What I learned is that we are always stronger than we know."
- Arnold Schwarzenegger

"A fit, healthy body -
that is the best fashion statement."
- Jess C. Scott

"The human body is the best work of art."
- Jess C. Scott

"What's the whole point of being pretty on the
outside when you're so ugly on the inside?"
- Jess C. Scott

"Keep working hard toward
whatever goal you've set for yourself."
- Jen Selter

"No gym? No problem! Try outdoor workouts."
- Jen Selter

"You're not gonna get the butt you want by sitting on it!!"
- Jen Selter

"Our bodies are our gardens
- our wills are our gardeners."
- William Shakespeare

"Don't have the goal of looking like the latest airbrushed model
on the cover of a magazine or lingerie catalog.
Instead, focus on becoming the best *you* possible
and forget about trying to achieve some 'ideal image'
as dictated by society and the popular media."
- Nia Shanks

"Eat real food at least 90% of the time.
Real food = items such as grass fed meats, wild caught fish,
free range eggs, fruits, veggies, nuts and seeds."
- Nia Shanks

"Highlight and improve upon your natural abilities and talents.
Don't compare yourself to anyone else."
- Nia Shanks

"It's more important that you develop habits
that are easy to maintain over a longer period of time
as opposed to employing a drastic change overnight."
- Nia Shanks

"Train because you love your body.
Not because you hate it.
Always have positive thoughts to fuel your workouts."
- Nia Shanks

"Give a man health and a course to steer,
and he'll never stop to trouble
about whether he's happy or not."
- George Bernard Shaw

"Use your health, even to the point of wearing it out.
That is what it is for.
Spend all you have before you die;
do not outlive yourself."
- George Bernard Shaw

"We don't stop playing because we grow old;
we grow old because we stop playing."
- George Bernard Shaw

"If a child in its first thousand days
- from conception to two years old
does not have adequate nutrition,
the damage is irreversible."
- Josette Sheeran

"Because of physicians' limited medical training,
rarely do we have the option to learn about
the true cause of disease.
And yet it is possible to prevent disease
and emotional breakdown."
- Bernie S. Siegel

"I began to realize a patient's beliefs
were more important than the diagnosis."
- Bernie S. Siegel

"If you talk to your body, it will listen."
- Bernie S. Siegel

"I know patients who bring a dozen roses to the doctor's office.
And, boy, the next visit, nobody forgets that.
You come in and hey -
'Here's the lady who brought the roses'
vs. 'Here's the lung cancer'."
- Bernie S. Siegel

"Inspiration is the greatest gift because
it opens your life to many new possibilities.
Each day becomes more meaningful,
and your life is enhanced
when your actions are guided by what inspires you."
- Bernie S. Siegel

"I was not a typical surgeon, because I kept
trying to help my patients in nontraditional ways."
- Bernie S. Siegel

"Laughter is one of the best therapeutic activities
Mother Nature provides us with,
and it doesn't cost a cent."
- Bernie S. Siegel

"Monday morning syndrome -
named after the day in the week when people have
more heart attacks, suicides, strokes, and illnesses."
- Bernie S. Siegel

"Most of us never stop to consider our blessings;
rather, we spend the day only thinking about our problems.
But since you have to be alive to have problems,
be grateful for the opportunity to have them."
- Bernie S. Siegel

"One of the best ways to change is to act
as if you are the person you want to become.
When you behave as if you are a different person,
you change on a very basic level
- even your physiology changes.
When actors and actresses perform,
their body chemistry is altered by the roles they play."
- Bernie S. Siegel

"Parents, teachers, clergy and physicians
change lives with their words.
It is hypnotic for a child or patient
to hear an authority figure's words.
As I am always sharing, 'wordswordswords'
can become 'swordswordswords,'
and we can kill or cure with either words or swords."
- Bernie S. Siegel

"People can be talked into health or illness."
- Bernie S. Siegel

"Physicians are not taught how to communicate with patients.
Because of their fear of being sued,
they tell people about all the adverse side effects
of therapy and never mention the benefits."
- Bernie S. Siegel

"The need for encouraging more
of a mind-body-spirit approach
in medicine is still great, especially
in the training of medical professionals."
- Bernie S. Siegel

"Scientists have studied the effects of laughter on the body
and identified a number of physiological benefits.
Laughter increases activity in the immune system,
giving 'good' killer cells a boost, especially in their ability
to target viruses, some tumors, and cancer cells."
- Bernie S. Siegel

"The doctor I would want for myself or for anyone else
I cared about would be one who understands that disease
is more than just a clinical entity;
it is an experience and a metaphor,
with a message that must be listened to."
- Bernie S. Siegel

"The mind and body are not separate units,
but one integrated system.
How we act and what we think, eat, and feel
are all related to our health.
Physicians should be capable of teaching
this behavior to patients."
- Bernie S. Siegel

"Today we have studies documenting that
cancer patients who laughed or practiced
induced laughter several times a day
lived longer than a control group who did not."
- Bernie S. Siegel

"Whatever we imagine, and what we focus on,
sends a message to our body,
so when we draw healing images
our body follows through."
- Bernie S. Siegel

"When lifestyle counseling was incorporated into the
medical treatment plan for patients with advanced cancer,
their survival time doubled and their quality of life improved."
- Bernie S. Siegel

"When you love your life and body,
your body will do all it can to keep you alive."
- Bernie S. Siegel

"You can't control the world, but
when you control your thoughts, you bring order."
- Bernie S. Siegel

"Your thoughts and feelings
create your internal chemistry."
- Bernie S. Siegel

"He who laughs, lasts."
- Bobbie S. Siegel

"Do what will make you happy."
- Rose Siegel

"Don't have $100 shoes and a 10 cent squat."
- Louie Simmons

"Sickness is the vengeance of nature
for the violation of her laws."
- Charles Simmons

"A kid who moves is a kid who learns."
- Richard Simmons

"For my workout, I'm up at 4 am
I say my prayers, count my blessings,
and I work out right away. I just get it done."
- Richard Simmons

"If you pick up every other magazine, it is the peanut butter diet,
or the cabbage soup diet, and then you go to the radio and you
hear that you can drink some solution
and you will lose weight overnight.
It just does not work that way!"
- Richard Simmons

"I've always practiced this:
Love yourself. Move your body. Watch your portions."
- Richard Simmons

"I have rules about eating, exercising and
rules about staying positive.
And these rules are sacred to me."
- Richard Simmons

"No tricks, gimmicks, special pills,
special potions, special equipment.
All it takes is desire and will."
- Richard Simmons

"Our children are obese, either have or
being threatened by diabetes, high blood pressure,
high cholesterol, and not socially adjusting
properly to others because of a lack of fitness."
- Richard Simmons

"Right now many schools have no recess.
Most schools have no PE."
- Richard Simmons

"If you wake up deciding what you want to give
versus what you're going to get,
you become a more successful person."
- Russell Simmons

"I go to yoga every day.
I meditate every morning."
- Russell Simmons

"I try to do things that I think
are helpful to the environment,
to the animals, and to the planet."
- Russell Simmons

"I mostly eat healthy. I just do.
I'm not a vegan for health reasons -
although obviously I'm 20 pounds lighter than when I started.
I stayed 20 pounds lighter. I feel better.
My friends say I look better. All that's true.
But I'm a vegan for compassionate reasons."
- Russell Simmons

"You can learn to follow the inner self,
the inner physician that tells you where to go.
Healing is simply attempting to do more of those things
that bring joy and fewer of those things that bring pain."
- O. Carl Simonton

"The question you need to ask yourself is
not if you will heal, but how you will heal."
- O. Carl Simonton

"When you're depressed,
the whole body is depressed,
and it translates to the cellular level.
The first objective is to get your energy up,
and you can do it through play.
It's one of the most powerful ways of breaking up
Hopelessness and bringing energy into the situation."
- O. Carl Simonton

"A doctor has to speak in positives.
If a doctor puts out negative energy,
the patients will take it in unconsciously."
- Stephen Sinatra

"The most important thing I can instill into the patient
is the belief that he or she can get well."
- Stephen Sinatra

"Eliminating grains and sugars from your diet
could be the number one most beneficial thing
you ever do for your health!"
- Mark Sisson

"If circumstances require that your sleep habits depart
from the earth's natural light and dark cycles,
make a strong effort to sleep with an eye mask
in a completely darkened room, since all of your skin cells
are sensitive and responsive to light - not just your eyes."
- Mark Sisson

"Our government's laws, subsidies, and diet education efforts
(grain-based USDA food pyramid, anyone?)
are seemingly driven more by lobbyists for the
beef, grain, and dairy industries than by unbiased
scientific evaluation and concern for human health."
- Mark Sisson

"Reduced Disease Risk Factors:
Ditching grains, sugars, other simple carbs,
and processed foods, especially 'bad fats' (trans and partially-
hydrogenated), will reduce your production of hormone-like
messengers that instruct genes to make
harmful pro-inflammatory protein agents.
These agents increase your risk for arthritis, diabetes,
cancer, heart disease, and many other
inflammation-related health problems."
- Mark Sisson

"Studies suggest that overweight kids are highly likely
to become overweight adults and consequently suffer
from serious health problems and life-threatening diseases."
- Mark Sisson

"The profound psychological benefits of play
are integral to healthy cultures,
communities, and individuals, including a
direct relationship to work productivity.
Engage in some unstructured outdoor physical exertion
each day to counter the negative effects
of a sedentary, technological existence."
- Mark Sisson

"Those who do not find time for exercise
will have to find time for illness."
- Edward Smith Stanley

"Have you ever noticed how there is always some new food
that is being 'discovered' for its mystical healing properties?
Every year it seems like there is another fad food that people
will flock to for a little while before they go back to eating
the way they have all their lives."
- Kimberly Snyder

"How close is the food to its natural state?
What sort of process did it undergo to wind up
in that package at the grocery store?"
- Kimberly Snyder

"I believe the word 'health' is synonymous with the word beauty.
My definition of beauty is that it's deep, lasting, and magnetic,
and it grows from the inside out."
- Kimberly Snyder

"That step of picking up your own food will
cut out more and more processed foods."
- Kimberly Snyder

"We are the only species on earth that
not only refuses to give up milk
but furthermore insists on drinking the milk of another species.
No adult cows ever drink milk, and adult humans are certainly
not meant to be drinking it, either!
As is always the case, when we go against nature's laws,
we suffer the consequences."
- Kimberly Snyder

"Why is it that two people get coughed on
directly in the face (gross!) by the same person
on the subway, but only one person gets the flu?
Dr. Robert Young gives a great analogy to this by pointing out
that if you throw seeds on concrete, they cannot grow.
But if you throw the seeds on fertile soil, they grow and flourish.
And so it is with germs and sickness."
- Kimberly Snyder

"All those spices and herbs in your spice rack can do more
than provide calorie-free, natural flavorings to
enhance and make food delicious.
They're also an incredible source of antioxidants and
help rev up your metabolism and
improve your health at the same time."
- Suzanne Somers

"Browsing our local farmer's market is
one of my family's favorite weekend activities.
Make it a relaxing, healthful habit for your family,
and you'll reap the nutritional rewards."
- Suzanne Somers

"Clean, tasty, real foods do not come processed in boxes or bags;
they come from the earth, the sea, the field, or the farm."
- Suzanne Somers

"Every chemical that makes it into your bloodstream
- be it through your lungs, stomach, or skin
meets up with your liver at some point.
Since your liver is your body's best defense when it comes to
filtering out all those toxins, you need to treat it well."
- Suzanne Somers

"From middle age on, there's nothing more vital to your
health and weight control than building lean muscle mass,
and the only way that happens
is with weight training and exercise."
- Suzanne Somers

"I am healthy;
it is the greatest gift I have given myself."
- Suzanne Somers

"I am in control of how I age,
and I am in control of my health."
- Suzanne Somers

"I appreciate health care that gets to the root cause
of our symptoms and promotes wellness, rather than the
one-size-fits-all drug-based approach to treating disease.
I love maintaining an optimal quality of life - naturally."
- Suzanne Somers

"I do yoga three times a week, and I walk for a half hour every day.
In between, I get on the elliptical and my triple thigh trainer
- I really do use the Thighmaster!
- and do about 20 minutes on each of those.
I also walk up and down the stairs a lot."
- Suzanne Somers

"I'm going to live to be 110 years old!"
- Suzanne Somers

"It is a very brave choice to go against traditional medicine
and embrace the alternative route.
It's easier to try the traditional route and then,
if it fails, go to the alternatives,
but often it can be too late."
- Suzanne Somers

"Reduce the stress levels in your life through relaxation techniques
like meditation, deep breathing, and exercise.
You'll look and feel way better for it."
- Suzanne Somers

"The biggest myth about aging is
that we can't do anything about it.
That it's a road to being decrepit, frail, and sick."
- Suzanne Somers

"Throughout my life, I have tried to share my belief that
getting and staying healthy doesn't have to feel like work.
My life is not about deprivation;
I don't diet or slave away in a gym.
What I do is eat clean, nutritious, real food.
I enjoy delicious meals with healthy fats,
I eat until I am full and satisfied, and I remain thin."
- Suzanne Somers

"We stopped cleaning our houses with
lemon water and vinegar like our mothers did,
and we clean with chemicals.
We're breathing chemicals,
and then everyone wonders
why cancer is the biggest killer."
- Suzanne Somers

"Heart disease continues to be the number one killer;
cancer, the number 2 killer, not far behind.
The tragic aspect of these deadly diseases
is that they could all be cured,
I do believe, if we had sufficient funding."
- Arlen Specter

"I've been playing squash almost daily for 38 years."
- Arlen Specter

"The best way to reduce the cost of medical care
is to reduce the illness."
- Arlen Specter

"There's nothing more important than our good health
- that's our principal capital asset."
- Arlen Specter

"Those who think they have not time for bodily exercise
will sooner or later have to find time for illness."
- Lord Edward Stanley

"Looking good and feeling good go hand in hand.
If you have a healthy lifestyle, your diet and nutrition are set,
and you're working out, you're going to feel good."
- Jason Statham

"How to stand: Whether you are at work,
chatting with a friend in the grocery store,
or standing in attention, your basic set up is always the same:
feet straight, back flat, belly tight, head neutral,
and shoulders externally rotated in stable position.
Don't be that guy who stands with arms crossed,
shoulders rolled forward, back slouched, feet angled out."
- Kelly Starrett

"It's not enough to exercise.
You have got to sleep.
You have got to drink enough water.
You have got to develop a practice
around maintenance of your body.
You have got to learn how to move right."
- Kelly Starrett

"When you can, avoid sitting, or even open up a direct attack.
Set your phone or watch timer to go off every hour
so that you get up out of your chair, mobilize for a minute or two,
and then (if you have to go back to sitting)
sit down with your butt and stomach muscles
turned on and engaged. "
- Kelly Starrett

"I grow my own vegetables and herbs.
I like being able to tell people that the lunch
I'm serving started out as a seed in my yard."
- Curtis Stone

"When I'm on the road, I tend to use hotel gyms.
When I'm home in L.A., I like to hike and hit the surf.
All in all, I try to keep a balanced diet and exercise routine,
which has stood me in good stead to date."
- Curtis Stone

"You've got to set yourself up to be as healthy as you can.
The thing we tend to do is when it gets to be a bit too hard,
actually opt out for the absolute worst option.
For example, if you're in a rush in a morning and you feel like
you don't have time to make breakfast, you skip it."
- Curtis Stone

"Deprivation doesn't work for me, and research shows
it doesn't work for most other people, either."
- Travis Stork

"Every time you sit down to eat,
you are making a life-changing decision.
You are deciding how well you want to live.
You are deciding how long you want to live.
And you are deciding how good you want to feel,
today and for the rest of your life.
In fact, every time you even look at a piece of food,
you are gazing at the destiny of your health."
- Travis Stork

"Focus on flavor, because life is too short to eat tasteless food!"
- Travis Stork

"No matter how bad your diet is,
no matter how much excess weight you're carrying around,
no matter how many food-related mistakes
you've made in the past, you can start fresh now."
- Travis Stork

"The biggest emergency in ERs across the United States
is the food we willingly, knowingly, happily choose to eat."
- Travis Stork

"Cardio is the easiest way to get us off our ass
and get our heart rates elevated.
It's why the American Heart Association
recommends 30 minute walks."
- Rob Sulaver

"First and Foremost, our food should be healthy.
Food is medicine. It can kill. It can cure. It's THAT powerful."
- Rob Sulaver

"I'm not saying NEVER indulge.
I'm saying, indulge intelligently.
Ideal nutrition strikes a perfect balance of
short and long term satisfaction.
It's your body and you're gonna have to live in it tomorrow.
That's why optimal nutrition isn't perfect.
It's balanced: Usually awesome.
Sometimes guilty. Occasionally downright glutenous.
Make the right choice 85% of the time and you're
Well on your way to a solid nutrition plan."
- Rob Sulaver

"Our abs sit under our belly fat and the two aren't related.
You have your abs... and then you have you belly fat."
- Rob Sulaver

"The food we consume should make us strong, capable,
and energized for whatever we do."
- Rob Sulaver

"Why are vegetables so damn good for us?
The vitamins and minerals in vegetables
are exceptionally bioavailable.
That means our bodies are very suited to digest and utilize them
('it's not what you eat, it's what you absorb.')
The phytochemicals in vegetables are also powerful anti-oxidants
and have a strong influence on our hormones.
They suppress cancer development,
protect our cell's DNA and stimulate enzymes
that help our body fight disease."
- Rob Sulaver

"Good health and good sense are two of life's greatest blessings."
- Publilius Syrus

"If you're capable of sending a legible text message between sets,
you probably aren't working hard enough."
- Dave Tate

"I'm just thankful for everything,
all the blessings in my life, trying to stay that way.
I think that's the best way to start your day and finish your day.
It keeps everything in perspective.
- Tim Tebow

"I rely on a lot of green drinks to get my vegetables."
- Tim Tebow

"Nutrition is also a valuable component that can help athletes
both protect themselves and improve performance."
- Bill Toomey

"Worrying about something is like paying interest
on a debt you don't even know you owe".
- Mark Twain

"A healthy outside starts from the inside."
- Robert Urich

"Cholesterol does not exist in vegetables.
Vegetables do not clog arteries."
- Jane Velez Mitchell

"According to exercise physiologists William McArdle
and Frank Katch, the average maintenance level
is 2,000 to 2,200 calories per day for women
and 2,700 to 2,900 calories for men.
Actual calorie expenditures can vary widely
and are much higher for extremely active people."
- Tom Venuto

"Burn the fat with training and
feed the muscle with nutrition."
- Tom Venuto

"Don't let your learning lead to knowledge,
let your learning lead to action."
- Tom Venuto

"The research shows that protein synthesis caps out around
30 or 40 grams and that spreading out your protein is better.
If you spread the protein evenly,
it usually averages out to about
25 to 30 grams per meal for women and
35 to 40 grams per meal for men during fat-loss programs
(maybe a little more for big, tall, or highly active people)."
- Tom Venuto

"There's no secret to getting started.
You simply decide and then take your first step.
With each subsequent step,
the next one becomes easier..."
- Tom Venuto

"What matters most is your ratio of muscle to fat
- your body composition.
With this distinction in mind,
losing weight should not be your only goal.
Your main focus should be
burning the fat and keeping the muscle."
- Tom Venuto

"Your mission is to find that 'sweet spot' in the middle where
intensity times duration yields the highest calorie burn.
I believe that sweet spot - which provides
both efficiency and effectiveness
is around 20 to 30 minutes of high-intensity cardio
or 40 to 45 minutes of moderate-intensity cardio."
- Tom Venuto

"Every day is game day. Prepare for it.
Fuel for it. Train for it. Rest for it."
- Mark Verstegen

"Happiness cannot be traveled to, owned,
earned, worn or consumed.
Happiness is the spiritual experience of living every minute
with love, grace, and gratitude."
- Denis Waitley

"You know, all that really matters is
that the people you love are happy and healthy.
Everything else is just sprinkles on the sundae."
- Paul Walker

"People who laugh actually live longer than those who don't laugh.
Few persons realize that health actually varies
according to the amount of laughter."
- James J. Walsh

"According to Ernest Wynder of the Sloan-Kettering Institute
for Cancer Research in New York, the time has come when
one can exterminate this kind of cancer with the help
of the active groups of the respiratory enzymes."
- Otto Warburg

"Nobody today can say that one does not know
what cancer and its prime cause may be.
On the contrary, there is no disease
whose prime cause is better known,
so that today ignorance is no longer an excuse
that one cannot do more about prevention.
That prevention of cancer will come there is no doubt,
for man wishes to survive.
But how long prevention will be avoided depends
on how long the prophets of agnosticism
will succeed in inhibiting the application of
scientific knowledge in the cancer field.
In the meantime,
millions of men must die of cancer unnecessarily."
- Otto Warburg

"I made a commitment to completely cut out
drinking and anything that might hamper me
from getting my mind and body together.
And the floodgates of goodness have opened upon me
- spiritually and financially."
- Denzel Washington

"Fitting a walk into a busy life can be challenging,
so I suggest walking rather driving to work
or to run errands as often as you can -
in other words, think of walking as alternative transportation."
- Andrew Weil

"Gardening is not trivial. If you believe that it is,
closely examine why you feel that way.
You may discover that this attitude has been
forced upon you by mass media
and the crass culture it creates and maintains.
The fact is, gardening is just the opposite -
it is, or should be, a central, basic expression of human life."
- Andrew Weil

"Human bodies are designed for regular physical activity.
The sedentary nature of much of modern life probably plays
a significant role in the epidemic incidence of depression today.
Many studies show that depressed patients who stick
to a regimen of aerobic exercise improve as much
as those treated with medication."
- Andrew Weil

"I am a particular fan of integrative exercise
- that is, exercise that occurs in the course of
doing some productive activity
such as gardening, bicycling to work,
doing home improvement projects and so on."
- Andrew Weil

"I have argued for years that we do not have
a health care system in America.
We have a disease management system -
one that depends on ruinously expensive drugs and surgeries
that treat health conditions after they manifest
rather than giving our citizens simple diet, lifestyle
and therapeutic tools to keep them healthy."
- Andrew Weil

"It does kids no favors,
and sets them up for a potential lifetime
of poor health and social embarrassment,
to excuse them from family meals of real food.
Everyone benefits from healthy eating,
but it is particularly crucial at the beginning of life."
- Andrew Weil

"Routines may include taking a warm bath
or a relaxing walk in the evening,
or practicing meditation/relaxation exercises.
Psychologically, the completion of such a practice
tells your mind and body that the day's work is over
and you are free to relax and sleep."
- Andrew Weil

"Studies have shown that people who are physically active
sleep better than those who are sedentary.
The more energy you expend during the day,
the sleepier you will feel at bedtime."
- Andrew Weil

"Technology has a shadow side.
It accounts for real progress in medicine,
but has also hurt it in many ways,
making it more impersonal, expensive and dangerous.
The false belief that a safety net of
sophisticated drugs and machines stretches below us,
permitting risky or lazy lifestyle choices,
has undermined our spirit of self-reliance."
- Andrew Weil

"The World Health Organization has recognized acupuncture
as effective in treating mild to moderate depression."
- Andrew Weil

"A man's health can be judged by which he takes
two at a time - pills or stairs."
- Joan Welsh

"A vigorous five-mile walk will do more good
for an unhappy but otherwise healthy adult
than all the medicine and psychology in the world."
- Paul Dudley White

"As a society, we have become so sick, weak, and broken,
we accept the abnormal as normal."
- Robb Wolf

"Despite the hype and promises, most supplements fail
to deliver much of anything."
- Robb Wolf

"Exercise is important, but diet is critical."
- Robb Wolf

"Fitness, like food, family, and friends, should be fun
and support your life, not take from it."
- Robb Wolf

"If you are concerned about skin cancer
because of this sun exposure,
keep in mind, safe, incremental sun exposure
(not burning your skin)
decreases your likelihood of developing a host of cancers far more
than it increases your likelihood of developing skin cancer."
- Robb Wolf

"Improved sleep is the most powerful thing folks can do
for their performance, health, and longevity."
- Robb Wolf

"It is worth noting, power is the physical attribute
that deteriorates fastest with age.
But it is also the fitness component
that gives us the greatest rewards if
we diligently train it throughout life."
- Robb Wolf

"The interior of the store (grocery) is your foe,
unless your buying detergent, coffee, or cat litter."
- Robb Wolf

"The United States is in a health care crisis, the economy is shaky,
and the government subsidizes the production of corn,
making high-fructose corn syrup cheaper than dirt.
Processed food manufacturers make crap foods that are
making us sick, diabetic, and dead too early.
The government subsidizes the development
of statins and a host of drugs
to manage the diseases that are a direct outgrowth
of the processed foods they are subsidizing!"
- Robb Wolf

"We were told to cut fat, increase 'complex carbs',
and all would be well.
That is true if you are in the business of coronary artery bypass,
statins, diabetes meds, or gastric bypass."
- Robb Wolf

"Worst-case scenario:
You spend a month without some foods you like.
Best-case scenario:
You discover you are able to live healthier and
better than you ever thought possible."
- Robb Wolf

"Trans fats ruin liver function.
They wreak havoc on blood lipids.
They destroy insulin sensitivity."
- Robb Wolf

"The athlete who says that something can't be done
should never interrupt the one who's doing it."
- John Wooden

"I'm killing two birds at once, so to speak.
Animal-based food kills people.
This way, by going vegan... we get healthy and save animals.
I'm being selfish, too, because if I can get my employees healthier,
we cut down on sick days and gain more productivity."
- Steve Wynn

"And when I started running, I started dreaming.
It couldn't be helped. The mind works as hard
as the body does during exercise.
It knows its role during those lonely interludes
- to inspire, analyze, and fantasize."
- Bart Yasso

"Running is about acceptance - of yourself and others.
When you're out on the trail sweating, it doesn't matter
if the guy or gal next to you works at a fast food joint or is CEO.
It's doesn't matter what color they are, or how old they are,
or what religion they practice, if any."
- Bart Yasso

"Running isn't about how far you go,
but how far you've come."
- Bart Yasso

"I know I feel more like myself when I run,
even if it's only a few miles,
or at least I feel like the self I like best.
Running inspires creativity, relieves stress,
and gives us insight into ourselves and the world,
making the human condition more tolerable."
- Bart Yasso

"The single biggest mistake that most beginners make is putting 100% of their effort into the positive (concentric) part of the rep, while paying no attention to the negative (eccentric) segment."
- Dorian Yates

"Running has the power to change your life.
It will make you fitter, healthier, even happier."
- Selene Yeager

"Education NOT Medication!"
- Robert O. Young

"Exercise your freedom to make healthy choices
and to take back your health."
- Robert O. Young

"Grow What You Eat and Eat What You Grow."
- Robert O. Young

"Health Care NOT Sick Care!"
- Robert O. Young

"It's no big secret that an alkaline lifestyle can do wonders
- from helping you lose weight and making sure you stay healthy.
The alkaline diet is so effective that
even celebrities have committed to it."
- Robert O. Young

"Once you know and believe that over-acidity
causes every disease and most dis-ease,
then to ignore that fact is a form of suicide.
When you eat poorly,
you pull the trigger every day of your life,
and eventually the gun fires.
The bullet might hit you square in the head
like a massive heart attack,
or it may kill you more slowly like a cancer,
or it may simply put you in a fog for the next 15 years
like Alzheimer's or dementia."
- Robert O. Young

"The blood never lies."
- Robert O. Young

"The body runs on electrons NOT calories."
- Robert O. Young

"The fish is only as healthy as the water it swims in.
If the water is clean YOU DO NOT GET SICK!"
- Robert O. Young

"Action conquers fear."
- Pete Zarlenga

"30 minutes a week of slow-motion weight training
burns more calories than regular-pace lifting
and is enough to get - and stay - in shape."
- Adam Zickerman

"If you do sit-ups quickly,
you're working off momentum,
but if you do them incredibly slowly,
you'll use nearly 100 percent
of your abdominal muscle fibers."
- Adam Zickerman

"We all know how important eating breakfast is,
but a lot of us neglect it."
- Adam Zickerman

"Working more muscle means burning more calories."
- Adam Zickerman

"A good laugh and a long sleep are
the best cures in the doctor's book."
- unknown

"An apple a day keeps the doctor away!"
- unknown

"Eat less, taste more."
- unknown

"He who takes medicine and neglects to diet
wastes the skill of his doctors."
- unknown (Chinese Proverb)

"If you always do what you've always done,
you will always be where you've always been
... Push through!"
- unknown

"Racing isn't about running until you're tired.
Racing is about running after you're tired."
- unknown

"The more you eat, the less flavor;
the less you eat, the more flavor."
- unknown (Chinese Proverb)

"There will come a day when you can no longer run...
Today is NOT that day!"
- unknown

Epilogue

You may be surprised about the people or quotes that were missing from this book. Part of the reason was to keep the book fairly short and also so the <u>end</u> of this book could be the <u>beginning</u> for you to keep reading even more health quotes. Perhaps you start your own collection of quotes that have a personal meaning and inspire YOU? You'll also notice a few quotes from us. We figured why not share a few thoughts or ideas we came up with and plant the seed that YOU too have probably at one time or another come up with some profound thoughts of your own. Why should other people be the only ones who come up with quotes? The next time you come up with a clever thought or saying, write it down and put some quotation marks around that idea or thought. Then share YOUR new quote with other people! If you come up with any really great quotes, please share them with us and we just might add them to one of our next books!

100% TOTAL SATISFACTION GUARANTEE:

If for ANY reason you are not 100% satisfied with the book or DVD you purchased, just send the product back along with receipt (or proof of payment). We will gladly refund 100% of your money, no questions asked!

Nemours Marketing, Inc.
7531 Azurebrook Court
Winter Park, FL 32792
info@NemoursMarketing.com
Tel: (407) 738 - 1608

www.ingramcontent.com/pod-product-compliance
Lightning Source LLC
Chambersburg PA
CBHW071153290526
45787CB00001BA/314